DIABETES RISING

Foreword by Zachary T. Bloomgarden, MD

DAN HURLEY

DIABETES
RISING

HOW A RARE DISEASE BECAME A MODERN
PANDEMIC, AND WHAT TO DO ABOUT IT

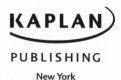

PUBLISHING

New York

© 2010 Dan Hurley

Published by Kaplan Publishing, a division of Kaplan, Inc.
1 Liberty Plaza, 24th Floor
New York, NY 10006

Printed in the United States of America

10 9 8 7 6 5 4 3 2

Library of Congress Cataloging-in-Publication Data

Hurley, Dan, 1957–
    Diabetes rising : how a rare disease became a modern pandemic, and what to do about it / by Dan Hurley ; with a foreword by Zachary Bloomgarden.
        p. ; cm.
    Includes bibliographical references and index.
    ISBN-13: 978-1-60714-458-8 (alk. paper)
    ISBN-10: 1-60714-458-1 (alk. paper)
    1. Diabetes—Epidemiology. 2. Diabetes—Etiology. I. Title.
    [DNLM: 1. Diabetes Mellitus, Type 1—epidemiology—United States. 2. Diabetes Mellitus, Type 2—epidemiology—United States. 3. Diabetes Mellitus, Type 1—history—United States. 4. Diabetes Mellitus, Type 1—prevention & control—United States. 5. Diabetes Mellitus, Type 2—history—United States. 6. Diabetes Mellitus, Type 2—prevention & control—United States. 7. Risk Factors—United States. WK 810 H965d 2009]
    RA645.D5H87 2009
    362.196'462—dc22

                                                                                          2009029382

For Annie.

CONTENTS

FOREWORD

THIS IS A STUNNING BOOK about diabetes, a disease that embodies much of the disharmony threatening modern man, and that appears, in a complex fashion, to be built into our basic genetic structure.

All living beings require a source of energy. For animals, from the simplest unicellular creature to the multicellular, multiorgan human, glucose is in an important sense the major energy source. Each cell of our body requires glucose to function, and contains within it the complex metabolic machinery to store glucose and to use it. It should come as no surprise, then, that nature has evolved a myriad of approaches to carefully husband glucose, to make it available when needed for work and for stress, and to assure that levels of it never fall too low. Fewer natural controls, however, exist in the body to avoid the opposite problem: glucose levels that rise too high. In the course of evolution, excess glucose was vanishingly rare; animals in general, and humans in particular, almost never had to face the problem of too much food, and therefore too much glucose.

Man's conquest of nature, gaining what appeared to be an endless supply of fuel, has given us the paradox of diabetes. Every mammalian species studied can with relative ease be caused to develop the equivalent of what is now called type 2 diabetes, simply by supplying food of the sort we make available in "convenience" stores around every thoroughfare in the world. Curiously, the other common form of diabetes, type 1, also appears to be related to the stresses of the modern world, through a complex process, less well understood, by which the immune system mistakenly identifies as foreign the single hormonal apparatus responsible for lowering glucose levels, the beta-cell of the islet of Langerhans of the pancreas, with consequent disastrous outcome for the person involved. Is this caused by too little exposure to common infections of childhood, or too much exposure to processed food (or perhaps even cow's milk), or to environmental pollutants, or to abnormalities of vitamins or minerals, or to genetic imbalances, or to some complex of all of these?

Dan Hurley has given us an understanding of all of these threads, and many more, leading to the modern epidemic of diabetes, which either in overt or potential form now appears to affect as much as one-quarter of the world's adult population. He wrote this book, as he tells us, in part because he has for so many years struggled with his own type 1 diabetes. I know personally of his struggles, and his successes, as his physician for over 20 years.

For patients, family members, physicians, and those simply interested in learning more about a disease so closely linked to the rise of modern civilization, *Diabetes Rising* offers not just a thorough background, but the hint of an "out of the box" approach to how we can treat and prevent diabetes. If the genesis of diabetes is based not only on our biochemistry, but also on our society and our approach to the environment, then the successful treatment and prevention of the disease will come not just from the hand of the physician, but from a partnership of governments, businesses, and concerned human beings who endeavor to put us more in harmony with our basic developmental needs.

As I read the manuscript, I found myself concurring with Dan, frequently saying, "Yes, this is how it happens," even if we do not yet have all the answers for how to fix the problems he spotlights. Kelly West, who many consider the father of diabetes epidemiology, wrote more than three decades ago in his classic book *Epidemiology of Diabetes and Its Vascular Lesions* about how simple it would be to prevent diabetes, by enjoining all people at risk to diet and to exercise regularly. So simple, yes, but do we know how to achieve this? Only with creative thinking of the sort Dan Hurley gives us in *Diabetes Rising* can we meet the global challenge of diabetes—with better understanding of the disease itself, and with impartial scrutiny of our latest theories, some of which may well prove as flawed as those from the past. Together, then, science and society can learn how to stabilize, perhaps improve, and hopefully reverse the rising threat of diabetes.

July 11, 2009

Zachary T. Bloomgarden, MD
Editor, *Journal of Diabetes*
Clinical Professor, Mount Sinai School of Medicine

PROLOGUE

T WELVE MILES WEST OF Boston lies its wealthiest, and seemingly healthiest, suburb. Along its winding, wooded roads, one can find a private tennis club, two golf clubs (including the 115-year-old Weston Golf Club and the nationally known Pine Brook Country Club), 13 soccer fields, and 19 baseball diamonds—and not a single fast-food restaurant. Established in 1713, the town has the highest median household income in Massachusetts, as well as the state's best public school system, according to *Boston* magazine. Its recreation department offers nearly 500 classes a year in yoga, karate, gymnastics, swimming, fencing, basketball, Pilates—even tap dancing. David Ortiz and Kevin Youkilis of the Boston Red Sox live there. Ray Allen of the Celtics lives just over the town line. The scent of overripe apples fills the air in the autumn, when tourists drive past the town's old stone walls and buy pumpkins from its roadside stands. Storybook beautiful, Weston is the kind of place where parents dream of raising their children.

So it took 41-year-old Rikki Conley by surprise when, early on the morning of September 17, 2007, she heard that another child in town might have the same rare, incurable, life-threatening illness that both of her young daughters, Ashley and Kelley, had been battling for years: type 1 diabetes mellitus—formerly known as "childhood onset," "insulin-dependent," or "juvenile" diabetes.

"That's ridiculous," Rikki thought to herself while speaking on the telephone to the mother of Kelley's best friend.

No other children in the elementary school that Kelley and Ashley attended had diabetes; the school nurse there had never before treated the disease, and had to learn everything from scratch. In fact, Rikki had to drive to other towns to attend coffees for parents of diabetic children hosted by the Juvenile Diabetes Research Foundation. So the idea that Kelley's best friend's brother, Gus, could now have it too—especially since the two families were so friendly, having occasionally gotten together for dinner or swimming—struck Rikki as simply impossible. And the pretty blue-eyed mom with honey-blond hair had as good a grasp of such things as any non-expert; after all, her husband, Kevin, was chairman of the board of the Joslin Diabetes Center, perhaps the most famous diabetes treatment and research institution in the world.

But here was Gus's mother, Ann Marie Kreft, calling her at 6:30 on a Monday morning.

"He had to go to the bathroom every fifteen minutes this weekend," Ann Marie said of her seven-year-old son, citing one of the cardinal symptoms. "Last night I saw him holding a water bottle under the faucet and then guzzling it. He's even started wetting the bed."

"I'll come right over and do a blood-sugar test," Rikki said calmly, now convinced that Ann Marie's suspicions weren't so groundless.

Within minutes of getting off the phone with Rikki, Ann Marie saw Gus wander out of his bedroom in his "bug" jammies, the ones with drawings of bugs all over them. By the time they made it down to the kitchen, Rikki was already pulling up in her minivan. Ann Marie's husband, Tim, was fixing breakfast for Gus, his older sister, and younger brother.

"What's Mrs. Conley doing here?" Gus asked when Rikki walked in.

"She brought Kelley's check," Ann Marie answered, using the Conley family's term for a blood-sugar meter. "She needs to do a check on you."

Rikki pricked his finger with a spring-triggered device and squeezed it for a drop of blood. She blotted it onto the end of an inch-long plastic strip protruding from the hand-held device that was the size of a cell phone. After what seemed like three years to Ann Marie, Gus's number flashed on the device's screen. Normal would be under 120. Gus's number was 292.

"Is there somewhere you and I can go?" Rikki asked Ann Marie.

The two women walked into the adjoining dining room, closed the door, and cried in each other's arms for a couple of minutes while Tim continued fixing breakfast for the kids.

During the two-day span of Gus's hospitalization at Children's Hospital, the Boston institution affiliated with Joslin, Rikki remembered something: another child in town had been diagnosed with type 1 diabetes back in April. Six-year-old Grayson Welo was just one year younger than Gus. She attended a private school, so neither Rikki's nor Ann Marie's children knew her. But she lived right around the corner from Gus, just a two-minute walk away. *How weird is that?* Rikki thought.

Less than two months later, things got weirder. On November 6, another little girl, Natalia Gormley, was also diagnosed with the supposedly rare disease on her tenth birthday. She lived just a few blocks from Rikki. A school nurse asked Ann Marie to let her know if any other new cases were diagnosed.

They didn't have long to wait. In the third week of January 2008, Rikki's daughter Kelley heard from a friend at the stables where she went horseback riding that another kid, 12-year-old Sean Richard, was diagnosed with diabetes on January 16. He lived less than a mile from Ann Marie, in a house that faced her street. That made four cases in nine months.

Having worked years earlier for the Massachusetts Department of Public Health as a health educator, Ann Marie decided to email a few friends who still worked there as epidemiologists to see whether they thought the four new cases exceeded the expected number for a town as small as Weston. Maybe, maybe not, they wrote back. It was right on the edge.

Six weeks later, eight-year-old Finn Sullivan became the fifth case of type 1 diabetes diagnosed in Weston in less than a year. He lived on Ann Marie's block, just six doors down.

Not easily frightened, but now certain that something serious was going on in her neighborhood, Ann Marie emailed her epidemiologist friends again. This time they told her she needed to request an official investigation from the state health department. None of them was quite certain what a normal rate of diabetes diagnoses should be, but whatever was going on in Weston, it wasn't normal.

They put her in touch with Suzanne K. Condon, associate commissioner and director of Environmental Health at the Massachusetts Department of Public Health. Condon remembered Ann Marie from when she worked there and assured her that she would have her staff look into the matter. In fact, she told Ann Marie, Massachusetts had recently become one of the only states in the country funded by the Centers for Disease Control and Prevention to establish an Environmental Health Tracking System. Although the program was initially examining local rates of childhood asthma, it could just as well track type 1 diabetes in children on a town-by-town level. She promised to begin doing just that. In the meanwhile, according to the best estimates from the CDC, for every 100,000 children in a given area, about 19 new cases should be diagnosed each year. With about 3,200 residents under the age of 18 living in Weston, the CDC statistics would mean that fewer than one child per year should be diagnosed with the disease.

Two months later, on April 28, six-year-old Mya Smith became the sixth case diagnosed in 12 months. Although she lived just over the town line, in neighboring Bryn Mawr, Mya and her family lived within two miles of all the other cases.

Then, on Sunday, June 15, came the jaw-dropper, when 17-month-old Walker Allen was diagnosed. Two nights later, his father, Ray Allen, scored 26 points in game six of the NBA playoffs to give the Celtics their first championship in 22 years.

Not knowing where the Allens lived, Rikki joked sarcastically to a friend, "He probably lives in our neighborhood." In fact, he did—less than half a mile from Ann Marie. This brought to seven the number of children diagnosed with type 1 diabetes in the past 14 months, all living within the same two-mile radius.

The town's school nurses had never seen anything like it. Even though some of the kids were too young for school, and some went to a private school or lived over the town line, there were now eight children with type 1 diabetes attending Weston public schools, including those diagnosed in previous years. By comparison, during the 18-year span between 1978 and 1996, the nurses could not recall there ever being more than one or two at any time in the 2,300-student public school system. Some years there had been none. Type 1 diabetes, after all, was supposed to be rare. *Really* rare.

On July 7, author James S. Hirsch of Needham, Massachusetts, published an open letter of support to Ray Allen in the *Boston Globe*, noting that his seven-year-old son, Garrett, also had diabetes (as Hirsch had chronicled in his book *Cheating Destiny*). Ten days later, Ann Marie and her husband published a letter with Kathy Richard, Sean's mother, to share their concerns about what they perceived to be a local epidemic in Weston.

"Three out of five families with recently diagnosed children live near enough for Allen and his son, Walker, to stroll to our homes, and a short car ride could take them to an additional two homes," they wrote. "Something's not right here. The lack of a national or even statewide diabetes registry complicates monitoring efforts, and we know little about what causes Type 1 diabetes. But we do know that these many diagnoses, in this tight proximity in this short period, are way out of the norm. We would be grateful if a researcher tried to figure out what's going on."

Although Ann Marie was already in touch with Dr. Condon at the Massachusetts Department of Public Health, she hoped to hear from academic researchers at one of Boston's many colleges and universities. She did. But she also began receiving letters and phone calls from parents in nearby towns, who shared their concerns about local rates far exceeding both current national averages and historic experience.

In Concord—site of the Old North Bridge and Walden Pond, and one-time home to Ralph Waldo Emerson, Louisa May Alcott, Nathaniel

Hawthorne, and Henry David Thoreau—five children were diagnosed with type 1 diabetes during the 2007–08 school year.

In nearby Mansfield, a total of 18 kids in the school system had the disease, enough to spark a parents' meeting with nurses, administrators, and representatives of the American Diabetes Association on the evening of October 18, 2008.

In Sudbury, the number of diagnosed children in the school system stood at an astonishing 27.

And in the nearby town of Woburn—where industrial pollutants had been linked to many cases of childhood and adult cancers, resulting in the infamous lawsuit featured in the book and movie *A Civil Action*—seven children in a single elementary school of 225 students had type 1 diabetes just a few years earlier.

As her concerns grew along with media attention to her cause, Ann Marie—described in a *Boston Magazine* article as having "an Erin Brockovich vigor about her"—began searching the online chat groups on *www.childrenwithdiabetes.org*, a popular site for families affected by the disease. There she found a posting by Analisa Cleland of Littleton, Colorado, a suburb of Denver, who wrote that seven children with type 1 diabetes lived in her neighborhood, "all within walking distance of my house . . . It sure makes me wonder if something is up . . . I must watch too much TV, I'm picturing the CDC coming to investigate the high incidence of type 1."

From the western suburbs of Phoenix, Arizona, Kelly Lyon responded, "I always picture the CDC coming to our door too! We have a lot of cities outlying here in the Phoenix area that have schools with crazy amounts of Type 1."

A mother in Colorado wrote, "My daughter is one of 3 girls on her softball team that are Type 1!! That is scary since there are only about 20 girls. Something isn't right!!"

From Sterling Heights, Michigan, Melissa O'Neill wrote about the junior high school her son, Brendan, attended. "Brendan's junior high school has 800 kids," she wrote. "There are now six type 1 diabetics in his school. Another boy was just diagnosed last week and is in one of his classes."

And from northern Georgia, yet another mother wrote, "I travel 30 minutes to a support group for the west part of our county. I was amazed that [there] were several moms from elementary schools that [have] 7 kids at each school."

So it was from north to south, east to west: the same alarms were being rung, and the same questions being asked, by parents, school nurses, and people with diabetes. Were these clusters of type 1 just statistical flukes, or were they real? If real, was the increase happening in just a handful of unlucky towns, or in many towns and cities, and in every state? What dark force could be behind the rise of such a dreaded, lifelong, life-shortening disease? And what, if anything, could be done to reverse it?

TWO TYPES, ONE DISEASE, BOTH RISING

This book seeks to answer these and other fundamental questions about the epic rise of diabetes, in both of its two major types, and the monumental efforts already underway to reverse the decades-long trend that has transformed a rare ancient disease into the defining affliction of modern Western civilization.

Most of us know the conventional wisdom about diabetes. It's pretty simple:

Type 1 is rare and strikes out of the blue, due in part to a genetic risk, set off by perhaps a virus or some other kind of stress. To treat it, you take insulin, test your blood sugars, and carefully watch what you eat. Self-management is the key to good control.

Type 2 is far more widespread, and spreading fast along with America's waistline. It's caused by eating too much and exercising too little. To treat it, you eat less and exercise more. If that fails, you take pills and perhaps insulin. As with type 1, self-management is the key to good control.

It turns out that this conventional wisdom is mostly misleading, mistaken, or outdated.

Type 1, it's true, used to be rare. Today, however, it's about twice as common among children as it was in the 1980s, about five times more common than in the years following World War II, and perhaps ten times more common than 100 years ago, if early statistics are to be believed. Genes have not changed; lifestyle and environmental risk factors have. Part 2 of this book will explore what those risk factors are. Suffice it to say for now, that while Weston might have unique local factors pushing its recent outbreak, it is also emblematic in many ways of the new normal across the United States, and indeed around the world: how we live and play and work, and why that has made us so curiously susceptible to type 1 diabetes.

Type 2 is also rising, of course, but far faster than the rate of obesity. In fact, the rate of new type 2 cases has doubled in the past decade, according to the U.S. Centers for Disease Control and Prevention. Shockingly, the CDC now projects that 33 percent of all boys and 39 percent of all girls born in the year 2000 will develop type 2 in their lifetimes. That's more than one in three overall. For blacks and Hispanics, the projections are even worse, tipping to over half—53 percent—of all Hispanic women, meaning that more of them will eventually have diabetes than do not.

Already, many people are developing the disease long before middle age. At Children's Hospital in Cincinnati, the rate of new diagnoses of type 2 in adolescents grew tenfold between 1982 and 1994. More recently, in the five years between 2001 and 2006, the percent of adolescent girls receiving prescription medications for type 2 nearly tripled—*in just five years.* Reports of kids dying from diabetes have even made their way into medical journals. Dying of type 2 diabetes in childhood? That's like getting Alzheimer's disease in high school.

It is worth stepping back to look at the big picture and consider what an aberration the rise of diabetes is in modern medicine. By contrast, cancer death rates in the United States fell by 18.4 percent among men and by 10.5 percent among women between 1991 and 2005, according to the American Cancer Society. Heart disease death rates fell by just over 25 percent between 1999 and 2005, according to the American Heart Association. Deaths due to stroke are likewise way down. Even the percentage of Americans ages 70 and over with dementia (ranging from mild memory loss to full-blown Alzheimer's disease) fell by 29 percent between 1993 and 2002. Diabetes, it would seem, is going the wrong way down a one-way street.

But take another step back: diabetes is growing at epidemic proportions not only in the United States. Rather, it can be fairly called a global pandemic, afflicting every continent and nearly every country. Indeed, diabetes was called a pandemic in the title of a 2006 book chapter co-authored by Venkat Narayan, MD, who recently stepped down as the CDC's chief epidemiologist on diabetes, and Pina Imperatore, MD, PhD, who took over that position. Consider the evidence:

- According to Takashi Kadowaki, MD, PhD, professor of diabetes and metabolic diseases at the University of Tokyo, "There has been an explosive increase in the prevalence of diabetes in Japan. In 1955, there were 1 million people with diabetes. Now there are nearly 30 million."

- The minister of health of Mexico, José Ángel Córdova Villalobos, MD, says of his country, "We could be in bankruptcy soon if we don't handle the diabetes problem."

- India, with more people suffering from diabetes than any other country in the world, now has an estimated 40.9 million with type 2—twice as many as were counted 12 years earlier, but just over half the number expected by 2025.

- In Bangladesh, where over a million human beings died in a 1974 famine, 8.5 percent of adults are now estimated to have type 2 diabetes.

- China has an estimated 40 or 50 million citizens with diabetes, with another million diagnosed each year.

- Even in rural Africa, a 2008 study found, 3.9 percent of people over the age of 15 have diabetes.

In the words of Gojka Roglic, MD, a leading specialist in the spread of diabetes at the World Health Organization, "Diabetes is probably the only disease in the world that has not seen a decline in at least some countries in the past 30 years. This applies even to countries that have a problem with under-nutrition."

Now take one final step back and ask yourself: 88 years after the discovery of insulin, with all the dozens of pills available for type 2, all the high-tech treatments available for type 1, and the estimated $116 billion per year spent on the medical treatment of diabetes in the United States alone, why the heck do more people get diabetes, and more people die of it, each year?

I ask these questions with more than the usual curiosity of a medical journalist. I was diagnosed with type 1 more than 30 years ago, at the age of 18. My late father had type 2, my mother's mother had it, and one of my older brothers was recently diagnosed with type 2 as well. So when I read yet another article or book about how we diabetics should just try harder and test our blood sugars more often and try some nifty new diet, I know enough to say that surely there has got to be a better way.

I am happy to report, after spending over a year interviewing hundreds of physicians, researchers, and patients in the United States and abroad, and even participating in a clinical trial, that there is a better way. Flying under the radar of most observers, a number of revolutionary approaches are making quiet, dramatic gains toward preventing, curing, or significantly improving the treatment of diabetes. As we shall see in Part 3 of this book, none of them involves lecturing people about the need to eat less and exercise more. None of them requires diabetics to test their blood sugars more often. And none of them places the blame for the disease and its dire consequences in the laps of diabetics. Instead, an astonishing body of evidence has been built in support of an interlocking group of theories, provocative as they are disturbing, as to why both type 1 and type 2 are rising in lockstep and how we can, for the first time in history, prevent or cure both of them.

Diabetes Rising seeks to trace how we dug ourselves into this hole, and how leading researchers believe we might climb out. Although I will occasionally share my own experiences when they seem pertinent, this will not be another memoir of living with diabetes. Nor will this be a book of advice, tips, heartwarming inspiration, or recipes; there are hundreds of those in the realm of diabetes.

This, instead, is something that has been curiously lacking: a work of impartial investigation rather than inspiration—of description, not prescription; of journalism, not paternalism—about the millennia-long quest to understand and cure what many consider the most mystifying, annoying, fascinating, and maddening disease known to humanity. This is the story of how diabetes rose from obscurity, and how a relatively small number of passionate, smart scientists, advocates, and public-policy strategists are struggling against orthodoxy to bring it to its knees.

To appreciate just how bizarrely unnatural the current mushrooming of the disease has become, it is useful to go back to a time when doctors could go their entire careers without seeing more than a handful of cases, or any at all. Part 1 of this book will narrate the biography of a disease called diabetes: how it started small, and grew into a monster.

PART ONE

THE RISING

CHAPTER 1

Pissing Evil

From Ancient Times to the Discovery of Insulin

ONCE UPON A TIME, diabetes was rare.

Hippocrates, perhaps the most famous physician of ancient Greece, considered the "father of medicine," made no mention of diabetes. Over 500 years later, Galen, a Greek-born physician who rose to prominence in Rome, wrote: "It is a very rare disease, which I have observed only twice until now." Still, he knew that other physicians had called it "dropsy of the chamber pot" or "urinary diarrhea."

Galen had it right about the urination. The very word *diabetes* comes from the Greek, meaning "to pass through" or "siphon." Frequent and copious urination—not just feeling the frequent need to go, as men with enlarged prostates often do, but actually peeing like there's no tomorrow—has always been considered the hallmark of the untreated, or undertreated, disease. Although plenty of other disorders can cause it, excess urination is so commonly identified with diabetes that medical historians trace the very first printed reference to the disease back to an Egyptian medical text written in the year 1536 B.C., and now known as the Ebers Papyrus, simply because it offers a number of remedies "for correcting urine that (is in) excess." One such remedy:

Cyperus grass, 1; grass seeds, 1; root of bhh shrub, 1; beat into a uniform consistency (and) steep in sweet beer. A bowl of this is drunk, along with the dregs.

Or,

Another remedy that reduces urine when it is (too) plentiful: groats of wheat, ⅛; desert dates, ⅛; Nubian ochre, 1/32; water, 1/64. Soak in rainwater, strain; to be taken for four days.

And then there's the old standby:

Grass roots, ¼; grapes, ⅛; honey, ¼; juniper berries, 1/32; sweet beer, 17/32. Cook, strain; to be taken for one day.

Another prominent Greek physician, Aretaeus of Cappadocia, likewise considered diabetes a rare disease, saying it was "not one very common to man." His vivid description of the disease is the first in Western medical literature:

The patients never cease making water, but the discharge is as incessant as a sluice let off. The disease is chronic in its character, and is slowly engendered, though the patient does not survive long when it is completely established, for the emaciation produced is rapid, and death speedy. Life too is odious and painful, the thirst is ungovernable, and the copious potations are more than equaled by the profuse urinary discharge; for more urine flows away, and it impossible to put any restraint to the patient's drinking or making water. For if he stops for a very brief period, and leaves off drinking, the mouth becomes parched, the body dry; the bowels seem on fire, he is wretched and uneasy, and soon dies, tormented with burning thirst.

To the east, in India, piquant descriptions of diabetes also appeared in a Sanskrit medical text, the Sushruta Samhita, dated to the sixth century B.C. Calling it a "diseased flow of the urine," or *Prameha*, the surgeon Sushruta wrote: "It may be prognosticated that an idle man, who indulges in day sleep, or follows sedentary pursuits or is in the habit of taking sweet liquids, or cold and fat-making or emollient food, will ere long fall an easy victim to this disease."

He further writes of a type called *Kaphaja*, which can be diagnosed "by the fact of the urine being assailed by a swarm of flies, lassitude, growth of flesh (obesity), catarrh, looseness of the limbs, a non-relish for food, indigestion, expectoration of mucous [*sic*], vomiting, excessive sleep, cough and labored breathing." (Other ancient authors wrote of dogs and ants being attracted to the urine, all due to its sweetness.)

Although Sushruta states that the disease, when sufficiently advanced, is incurable, elsewhere he asserts that an herb called Silajatu "cures an attack" of diabetes "and enables the user to witness a hundred summers on earth, free from disease and decay." Each dose of this Silajatu, he goes on, "taken successively, adds a century to the duration of human life, while 10 doses extend it to a thousand years."

A TASTE OF HONEY

Some two millennia after Sushruta, London physician Thomas Willis offered treatments for diabetes that sound, to modern ears, no less ridiculous. The third chapter of his 1679 book *Pharmaceutice Rationalis* was entitled "Of the too much Evacuation by Urine, and its Remedy; and especially of the Diabetes or Pissing Evil, whose Theory and Method of Curing, is inquired into." In it, he offered such spice-rack remedies as cinnamon, rhubarb, gum "arabick," and, ironically enough, sugar.

Yet he professed little faith in such potions, writing: "It seems a most hard thing in this Disease to draw true propositions of curing, for that its cause lies so deeply hid, and hath its origine so deep and remote." And he was astute enough to be the first Western physician to emphasize the taste of diabetics' urine being "wonderfully sweet as if imbued with Honey or Sugar," which led to the medical term that has persisted to this day, *diabetes mellitus,* from the Latin for "honey-like." (How did Willis know what their urine tasted like? Physicians since medieval times had made the tasting of urine for diagnosis of diseases such a common practice that they were typically depicted in drawings of the era as holding a flask of the stuff.)

Willis asserted in his 1679 book that diabetes had by then become more common than it was in ancient times: "In our Age given to good fellowship and gusling down chiefly of unalloyed Wine; we meet with examples and instances enough, I may say daily, of this Disease." Yet by the time the next great treatise on diabetes was published, in 1798, it had again become so rare that after seeing a single case, the physician John Rollo wrote that he did not see another for 22 years, even though he had traveled widely in the intervening years, to America, Barbados, and England, as a physician for the English army. Rollo became curious enough that he wrote to other physicians, asking them to share their own case reports. His resulting book, *Cases of the Diabetes Mellitus,* was the first publication in history to prescribe a low-carbohydrate diet for the disease, advising that patients begin by eating only "animal" food (that is, meat), and then carefully adding vegetables unlikely to produce sugar in the urine. "The vegetable substances we have hitherto found the safest," he wrote, "are, broccoli, spinage [sic], cauliflower, cabbage, and lettuce." Modern advocates of low-carb diets would have no quarrel with Dr. Rollo's recommendations, nor with his honest assessment of the typical diabetic's response:

> We have to lament, that our mode of cure is so contrary to the inclinations of the sick. Though perfectly aware of the efficacy of the regimen, and the impropriety of deviations, yet they commonly trespass, concealing what they feel as a transgression

on themselves. They express a regret, that a medicine could not be discovered, however nauseous, or distasteful, which would supersede the necessity of any restriction on diet.

As accurate as were the descriptions of Dr. Rollo and his ancient predecessors, it is striking that none of them emphasized the chief predisposing risk factor that we all now associate with type 2 diabetes: excess weight. In fact, only one of the old medical texts even makes passing reference to weight: the Sushruta Samhita, as noted above, which states that one kind of diabetes, *Kaphaja,* is distinguished in part by "growth of flesh." Otherwise, the doctors of yore fall curiously silent on weight and obesity. True, they sometimes noted the risks of overindulging in sweets or starchy foods, but such habits are hardly synonymous with being overweight.

How are we to explain that a physician like Dr. Rollo, for all his powers of observation, was unable to put two and two together: that excess weight is the primary risk factor for diabetes, and so getting rid of the former should be the best way to cure the latter? Two possibilities jump out.

First, perhaps he and his predecessors saw only type 1 diabetes, which is not generally associated with being overweight. But to the contrary, nearly all the early descriptions of diabetes are plainly of type 2, involving adults, not children, whose symptoms typically came on slowly (as they often do in type 2), not quickly (as they almost always do in type 1). That is not to say that type 1 was utterly unknown, although physicians recognized no such distinctions. Dr. Rollo wrote that he had heard of a case of diabetes in a 12-year-old, which almost surely would have been type 1. And in 1810, the New York surgeon Valentine Mott published *An Account of an Extraordinary Case of Diabetes Mellitus,* involving a nine-year-old boy who died in a matter of weeks from the time Dr. Mott first saw him—this despite Dr. Mott's best efforts, which included bleeding the boy regularly, and prescribing him opium and arsenic.

The second possibility is that, because untreated diabetes causes weight loss (since the life-sustaining glucose is being peed out instead of used by the body), physicians were seeing patients whose weight, by the time they sought medical assistance, appeared anything but excessive. And indeed, sudden weight loss was described as a standard symptom of diabetes by physicians all the way back to Aretaeus.

But, then again, weight loss has long been seen as a symptom in all kinds of diseases, including cancer and tuberculosis—regardless of the person's weight at the onset of the illness. Thin people who developed diabetes or cancer got thinner, just as fat people did. The point is, being overweight was never seen as a risk factor for any of those illnesses.

I do not mean to suggest that physicians never saw any overweight people with diabetes. The perspicacious Dr. Rollo told of just such a patient of his: "Captain Meredith, of the Royal Artillery, being an acquaintance of mine . . . always had impressed me, from his being a large corpulent person, with the idea that he was not unlikely to fall into disease. On the 12th of June, 1796, he visited me, and . . . I was at once struck with the diminution of his size." But Dr. Rollo did not write that he had always suspected Captain Meredith would become diabetic, only that he would "fall into disease"—any of the many diseases even then associated with obesity, such as gout and heart disease.

We are faced with the mystery, then, that pre-industrial physicians like Dr. Rollo and Dr. Willis, straight back to Aretaeus, were generally talking about type 2, yet they never noticed that the leading risk factor for the disease is *obesity*. Rather than suspecting them of being dull-witted when it comes to something so obvious, we need to confront the more likely, and to our modern sensibility quite surprising, fact that most diabetics in those days simply did not weigh much more than the average person. Diabetes being so relatively rare in pre-modern times, what these physicians were apparently seeing, we can only assume, were those folks with the greatest inherent tendency—what we would now understand to be the most extreme genetic risk—toward developing the disease *at even a normal weight.* Remember: there were no bags of chips to be bought for 75 cents in those days, and no McDonald's restaurants to drive through; for that matter, there were no cars to drive. And so what diabetes developed was the very soul of the disease in its most basic form. Which permits us to infer that while diabetes is certainly exacerbated by weight, it is ultimately not caused by it.

But we are getting ahead of our story.

FIRST BREAKTHROUGH

In 1866, the year after the Civil War ended, New York City's death rate from diabetes was just 1.4 for every 100,000 residents. Two years later, when Charles B. Brigham wrote a prize-wining paper on diabetes while still a student at Harvard University, the disease was still so rare that he found only 40 reports of death attributed to it by Boston's city registrar in the 12 years between 1854 and 1866—fewer than four cases per year, on average. Although he knew of at least one infant who died of it, he judged that, on the whole, "the disease is one of middle age rather than of youth, and the maximum mortality is between the ages of twenty-five and sixty-five years."

Brigham made no mention of diabetics being overweight. While he quoted doctors who questioned the practicality of forcing diabetics onto a low-starch diet, he reported little doubt about the diet's efficacy (for those able to follow it). He went so far as to list the percent of starch to be found in fruits, vegetables, beers, and wine, and even discussed the merits of forced exercise.

As to the cause of the disease, he described various theories and observations, including cases in which it could be induced "by standing for a long time in cold water; and also those in which diabetes occurred in sailors who were exposed to wet and cold from shipwreck." In his view, however, "The immediate causes of Diabetes are nearly as obscure as [are] the remote [causes]."

The first true breakthrough in understanding the biological cause of diabetes, or at least one of the causes, came purely by accident. In 1889, the German scientists Oskar Minkowski and Joseph von Mering disagreed on whether pancreatic juices were necessary for fat absorption. They had no particular interest in diabetes, but to settle their debate they needed to remove the pancreas of a dog and see what happened to its ability to absorb fat. Once Minkowski had successfully completed the operation (which was a tricky enough procedure that many who had tried it before had mistakenly left behind a small portion of the pancreas), he noticed that the dog began peeing inordinately.

According to a popular version of what happened next, Minkowski's colleague, Bernhard Naunyn, then asked, "Have you tested the urine for sugar?" Minkowski replied that he had not. "Do it," Naunyn supposedly said. "For where the dog passes urine, the flies settle."

Yep, Sushruta's flies.

Good story, but Minkowski later denied that flies had ever been seen. Rather, he insisted, Naunyn had previously taught him to always test for sugar in the urine whenever he noticed that an animal was peeing a great deal. In any case, he did test for sugar, and he found it to be high. He then fully removed the pancreases of other dogs and found the same result. Loss of the pancreas, it was soon announced to great fanfare in medical journals, causes diabetes.

For the following two decades, a variety of researchers attempted the logical next step: removing the organ, grinding it up, and giving the extract to other de-pancreatized animals, whether by mouth or injection. The oral route brought no effect whatsoever, but injections of pancreatic extract did sometimes lower sugar levels in both animals and, then, in humans. However, they also caused severe inflammatory reactions toxic enough to kill. Leaders in the field soon passed judgment that whatever the pancreas did, injecting bits of it into the diabetic was a dead end.

Meanwhile, Dr. Frederick M. Allen began work on a different approach: starvation. In 1913, he published a report showing that diabetic cats and dogs subjected to a near-starvation diet lived far longer than those allowed to eat freely. Soon after he began advocating the treatment in humans, limiting not just the carbohydrates of diabetic patients but the fats and proteins too, an approach that was soon "heralded as the greatest step yet accomplished in the treatment of the disease," according to a 1920 report in the *New York Medical Journal*. He didn't quite starve the patients to death; actually, he starved them to life. He began by restricting all food until the person's urine became free of sugar, then allowed only as little as would remain compatible with sugar-free urine. Thus treated, even children who obviously had what we would now consider type 1 could survive, wraithlike, for years.

Allen's treatment was quickly picked up by Dr. Elliott P. Joslin, the Boston physician who in 1898 had opened the first medical practice devoted purely to diabetes, launching what would become the world-famous Joslin Clinic. But not all physicians were buying the tough approach championed by Allen and Joslin. "Individualizing is one of the mainstays of diabetes," wrote Dr. Henry S. Stark in that same 1920 issue of the *New York Medical Journal*, railing against physicians who "religiously proscribe sugar." (Stark also offered his thoughts on the use of opium for the disease, "the most frequently prescribed drug in the treatment of diabetes even today," he wrote. Although he soberly counseled against undue faith in its benefits, he pronounced that it did sometimes seem to help.)

THE RISE BEGINS

By the early 1920s, with the first pieces of the modern American lifestyle beginning to fall into place—the Model T rolling off Ford assembly lines, Charlie Chaplin starring in films, and Betty Crocker invented as a brand name for the company that would become General Foods—diabetes was recognized, for the first time in history, as being indisputably on the rise. "It is no exaggeration to assert that as a disease incidence diabetes will soon rank with tuberculosis and cancer in frequency and fatality," Dr. Stark wrote in his 1920 *New York Medical Journal* piece. "It has trebled itself in thirty years." And, not coincidentally, the subject of weight had at last come to the fore. "Obese and gouty subjects, likewise those who overeat," Dr. Stark wrote, "should be ever watchful of the disease."

Actually, Dr. Stark underestimated the extent of the increase in diabetes. Just look at the numbers, from 1866 to 1923:

- Whereas only 1.4 of every 100,000 New York City residents had died of diabetes back in 1866, by 1900 the toll had reached 10 of every 100,000.

- A decade later, the city's death rate from diabetes was 16 for every 100,000 residents.

- By 1923, it stood at 22.9 per 100,000—an astonishing 16 times higher (not 16 percent, but *1,600* percent) than it had been only two generations earlier.

According to Dr. Haven Emerson, who served as the city's health commissioner from 1915 to 1917, then as a delegate to the International Conference on the Classification of Causes of Death in 1920, and was appointed professor of preventive medicine at Columbia University's medical school in 1921, diabetes by then was most commonly seen among wealthy merchants, and was still rare among manual laborers. He considered it a disease of the rich, who could afford to eat as much as they liked and who liked to be seen as fashionably fat—visual evidence of their wealth.

So it was that a disease that had remained rare since the dawn of recorded history, and was still so as recently as the Civil War, was now commonplace, frequently cited as a cause of death or disability among leading figures of the day. On May 22, 1920, the Associated Press reported, Japanese emperor Yoshihito was suffering from it, and two months later, unable to speak clearly or attend state functions, he was rumored to be already dead of it (although he lived until 1926). A year later, in May of 1921, legendary union leader "Big Bill" Haywood was said to be ill with the disease, which contributed to his death in 1927. On February 18, 1922, Bethlehem Steel chairman Charles M. Schwab's 57-year-old brother died of diabetes at 3:30 P.M. in his room at New York City's Hotel Collingwood, leaving behind a wife and two children.

And then, on March 23, just over a month after Schwab's brother's death, the *New York Times* published a three-paragraph article on its front page under the headline "Canadian Doctors Report Discovery That Checks Diabetes." Researchers at the University of Toronto had discovered an "active pancreatic extract which it is hoped will prolong the lives of persons suffering from diabetes." Two young doctors, who the *Times* identified as "F. G. Branting and C. H. Best," had first prolonged the life of a diabetic dog 56 days beyond previous records. "Then," the report went on, "by injecting under the skin of seven human beings suffering from the disease a highly potent extract discovered through animal experimentation, a distinct improvement was brought about in the patients."

Unfortunately, false reports of cures for all kinds of diseases were common in those days, even in the most respected newspapers. In June of 1918, the *Times* reported on an Italian doctor's claim that he could cure tuberculosis with sugar. A headline in October of that year announced, "Insanity Due to Infected Teeth; Cures Follow Extraction."

As for diabetes, the *New York Times* published three articles, in 1912 and 1913, about curing diabetes with a kind of bacterium found in yogurt, and another in 1915 about curing it with baking soda. How much more credible this new report of an alleged cure might be, particularly after years of failure with pancreatic extracts, was anybody's guess.

LITTLE ISLANDS

By the time of the March 23, 1922, news report, Frederick Grant Banting—not "Branting," as the *Times* had misspelled it—was in despair, drinking himself to bed every night and all but pushed aside from

13

continuing work on the pancreatic extract, which, in any case, was no longer lowering sugar levels in diabetic animals or people. To top it off, according to historian Michael Bliss's definitive and engrossing book *The Discovery of Insulin,* Banting's longtime girlfriend, Edith Roach, had written to him on March 17 to say goodbye.

From the start, the young Canadian physician had been singularly unqualified to discover a cure for anything. Raised on a farm, with no advanced scientific degree and no experience in research, Banting had found himself back in July of 1920 struggling to find patients for his new medical practice in the small city of London, Ontario. That month he had earned a grand total of $4. He could not even afford to take Edith out to the movies. To earn a few extra dollars, he began that fall to teach a course in surgery and anatomy at the local university.

With no knowledge of diabetes beyond what he had learned in medical school, and having never treated a diabetic patient, Banting, then all of 28 years old, spent a few hours on the evening of October 31 preparing for a lecture he was to give the next day on carbohydrate metabolism. He then went to bed with a copy of the journal *Surgery, Gynecology and Obstetrics.* In it he happened across an article touching on the subject of his talk. "The Relation of the Islets of Langerhans to Diabetes with Special Reference to Cases of Pancreatic Lithiasis" described a case in which a blockage of the main pancreatic duct leading to a patient's stomach had resulted in an atrophy of nearly all the cells in the pancreas, except for the so-called islets of Langerhans.

First identified in 1869 by German scientist Paul Langerhans, who said they looked like "little islands" in the pancreas when viewed under the microscope, the islets had long been suspected as playing a special role in the development of diabetes. The novel finding in the article was that the patient, whose islets were the only tissue in the pancreas that had remained healthy, did not develop diabetes. Similar results had been previously observed when the pancreatic ducts were intentionally tied off by surgeons: minor stomach ailments, but no diabetes.

Setting the journal aside, Banting tried to go to sleep but found he couldn't. "I thought about the lecture and about the article and I thought about my miseries and how I would like to get out of debt and away from worry," he later wrote in his memoir. "Finally about two in the morning after the lecture and the article had been chasing each other through my mind for some time, the idea occurred to me that by the experimental ligation of the duct and the subsequent degeneration of a portion of the pancreas, that one might obtain the internal secretion free from the external secretion. I got up and wrote down the idea and spent most of the night thinking about it."

Banting had imagined a surgical work-around to the problem that had, he suspected, botched previous researchers' attempts to get whatever it is in the pancreas that prevents diabetes. Their injections of pancreatic extract, he reasoned, had contained not only the material from the islets of Langerhans but the digestive juices that are meant for the stomach, and that might destroy the good stuff coming from the islets. He would operate on a dog, tying off the ducts leading from its pancreas to its stomach, and then wait days or weeks for the backed-up pancreas to wither away—all, that is, except for its islets, still happily doing their thing. Then he would surgically remove the pancreas, with only its islets intact, isolate whatever magic stuff was inside them, and give it to a diabetic. *Voilà!*

As simple as the idea seemed in theory, Banting in fact had none of the necessaries, practical or intellectual, to act upon it. Completely ignorant of the many previous studies that had attempted to isolate whatever useful substance was coming from the pancreas, he also had no clue how to properly remove the pancreas of a dog to render it diabetic; how to identify the pancreatic ducts, much less tie them off; how to test for sugar in the blood and urine, in order to see what effect any injections might have; or even how to properly macerate and filter the degenerated pancreas in preparation for injecting it into a diabetic dog. Oh—and he had no lab, no dogs, and no money.

What Banting did have going for him was *desperation:* he needed to make a living. Also, he had a good deal of experience as a surgeon, having served in the Canadian Army Medical Corps on the front lines during World War I. And, perhaps not least of all, he had in fact stumbled upon a hell of a good idea, which apparently none of the experts had ever thought of or attempted.

The morning after his idea had come to him, he spoke to a professor at Western University, where Banting taught, but the professor said that someone else had probably already tested it, and in any case Western had no facilities for such experiments. He suggested that Banting talk to an expert on the subject, J. J. R. Macleod, a professor of physiology at the University of Toronto.

A week later, Banting showed up at Macleod's office. The senior professor at first listened attentively but then began shuffling through papers on his desk. Banting repeated his pitch, and this time Macleod sat back in his chair, closed his eyes in thought, and said that the idea was worth trying. However, he added, it would take months of work, and in all likelihood the results would turn out to be negative. But even a negative result would be worth achieving, Macleod said, to settle the matter once and for all of whether something within the pancreas could be found to treat diabetes. So if Banting wanted to come and give it a shot, Macleod told him, he was welcome.

Already deeply in debt, and reluctant to abandon his fledgling medical practice or his teaching job at Western University in order to pursue a theory that was likely to fail, Banting told Macleod that he'd think about it. Before heading home, he discussed the matter with Clarence L. Starr, the chief of surgery at Toronto's Hospital for Sick Children. In December, Starr wrote to Banting to say that Macleod thought it would be unwise for him to quit his work in London, but that if he wanted to spend a month or two of his next summer vacation on the experiment, he was welcome to use Macleod's laboratory. Banting waffled over the coming months, going so far as to apply to be the medical officer for an oil-exploration team heading up to the Northwest Territories. But when the job didn't pan out, he took the train for Toronto.

NEAR TOTAL FAILURE

On Tuesday, May 17, Macleod helped out for the first operation on a dog, a brown spaniel female, with medical student Charles Best serving as assistant. Having demonstrated the basic surgical techniques, Macleod then left Banting and Best to their own devices for the following procedures. By Saturday, they had operated on four dogs, all of whom died. By the end of the second week, seven of the ten dogs they had operated on were dead. By early July, 14 of 19 dogs were dead, and only two of the dogs whose pancreatic ducts had been tied were showing signs of the intended pancreatic degeneration. As Bliss describes it in his history, "The whole research program was not far from total failure."

But on Saturday, July 30, they decided to remove the shriveled pancreas of one of the surviving duct-tied dogs. Following the advice of Macleod, who had gone away for the summer on vacation to Scotland, they sliced up the pancreas, placed pieces of it into a mortar along with ice-cold salt water, then chilled the mortar until its contents were partly frozen. Using a pestle and sand to grind up the pancreas along with the salt water, they then filtered it through cheesecloth and blotting paper to get a pink liquid extract. They warmed it to room temperature and injected it into the vein of a white terrier whose pancreas had previously been removed and whose blood sugar was now at 200. An hour later, the dog's blood sugar fell to 120, then slowly went back up despite several other injections. By the next day, the dog was dead.

They tried again the following day on another de-pancreatized dog, one whose blood sugar was so high that it was lapsing into coma. After two injections, the dog was well enough to briefly stand and walk around, but it soon lapsed back into a coma and died. On Thursday, August 4, they began injecting their third de-pancreatized dog, a yellow collie. Now calling the extract "isletin," after the islets from which it came, they succeeded in keeping the collie alive through a series of injections for three days, until noon on Sunday. On August 11 they removed the pancreas of another yellow collie. Despite giving it injections made from whole pancreas, not the withered pancreas that Banting had thought necessary, the dog lived until the 31st.

In fact, as would eventually become apparent, Banting's original idea for tying off the ducts and getting the pancreas to shrivel up before using it had nothing to do with their initial success. The idea had merely gotten them going. Rather, it was Macleod's insistence on keeping the extract nearly frozen until it was filtered that proved essential, by preventing the digestive juices in the pancreas from destroying the "isletin," and removing most of the contaminants.

By the time Macleod returned from his vacation, on September 21, Banting was confident enough in his results to demand a modest salary (he had been earning nothing until then) as well as slightly improved working conditions in the laboratory. When Macleod hesitated, Banting threatened to leave the University of Toronto for another institution. Macleod relented, and the work went on.

Following Macleod's instructions, Banting and Best began performing more tests on the dogs, before and after treatment, to prove beyond a doubt that the reduction in blood-sugar levels following injection of the isletin could not be explained by other factors, such as simple dilution of the blood from the injections. By late November, they submitted a paper on their results so far to the *Journal of Laboratory and Clinical Medicine,* which accepted it. By December, with the help of biochemist James B. Collip, they began using alcohol rather than water for preparation of the extract, which appeared to improve its purity.

THE FIRST PATIENT

By January 11, 1922, the group felt ready to try giving an injection of isletin to a human. Fourteen-year-old Leonard Thompson was selected. Weighing 65 pounds when he had been admitted to the Hospital for

Sick Children a month earlier, the boy had survived on Dr. Allen's starvation diet for more than two years since developing diabetes. But the isletin proved a failure. Although his blood-sugar level briefly declined from 440 to 320 after receiving 15 cubic centimeters of it, he also developed an abscess at the site of one of his injections and felt no less sick. His doctors concluded that, in his dire condition, he could not risk another injection.

Collip went back to work on improving the purity of the extract, eventually finding that a solution of 90 percent alcohol was best for drawing out the impurities. At 11 A.M. on Monday, January 23, they resumed injecting Leonard Thompson, this time using Collip's extract. In a day his blood-sugar level fell from a dangerously high 520 to a nearly normal 120, and he soon reported feeling better and stronger. Six more patients were treated at the hospital, all responding positively.

On January 27, a dog named Marjorie, whose pancreas had been removed back on November 18, was still alive after 70 days, thanks to continued injections. On that day, they decided to chloroform and kill the dog in order to reserve the limited supply of isletin. (Then, as now, some people opposed the killing of animals in research, no matter the potential benefits to people; known as "antivivisectionists," they often protested on the sidewalks outside the university's laboratories.)

As heady as one might think these days would have been for Banting, in fact he was miserable. Prone to fits of rage and despair, jealous of his colleagues' contributions and paranoid that they would rob credit for the discovery, he felt sidelined by the increasingly technical biochemical work in which Collip and Macleod were engaged. The "experts" were taking over, leaving Banting and Best as little more than assistants. Banting still had no formal appointment at the university, no certain future there, and was not even credentialed to work as a physician at the Hospital for Sick Children. Indeed, some at the hospital said he was not qualified to treat the disease for which he had played such a pivotal role in finding a life-saving treatment.

Under unrelenting pressure for months, now drinking heavily in his apartment every night, he was not even consulted on the writing of the next medical paper. Just around this time, Edith broke up with him, and production of isletin came to a crashing halt. Collip's new extraction process, which he had worked so hard to perfect, suddenly stopped working. Somehow he had gotten mixed up on his own method.

It was just then, in mid-March of 1922, that the *New York Times* published its three-paragraph article about their discovery.

Of course, everything worked out in the end. Banting and colleagues resolved the challenges with extraction, changed the name from isletin to "insulin" (from the Latin word for "island"), and brought forth to an amazed and thankful public the first effective drug for diabetes. Virtually overnight, emaciated diabetic children who had been clinging to life by the thread held out by Allen's and Joslin's starvation treatment were able to put on pounds and regain their strength. With the Eli Lilly Company working to crank up production to an industrial scale, Banting appeared on the cover of *Time* magazine and received, along with Macleod, the Nobel Prize in medicine in 1923 (they split their prize money with Best and Collip).

That spring, Dr. Joseph Collins published an article in the *Times* under the headline "Diabetes, Dreaded Disease, Yields to New Gland Cure." He called diabetes only the latest illness to succumb to science. "Its conquest is a feather in the cap of science," Dr. Collins wrote.

But insulin wasn't a cure, only a treatment, and its discovery wasn't the end of the story, only the dawn of a new phase. Then as now, the fact that it required daily injections with a needle (in those days, fat hypodermics that needed to be sterilized in boiling water after every use and sharpened by hand) was hardly a minor stumbling block. Of course, for desperate parents otherwise left to watch their children slowly starve to death in the clinics of Allen or Joslin, insulin was a true medical miracle—if, that is, they could get their hands on any, and if they could afford it. But as another headline in the *Times* stated on July 8, 1923, "Insulin, New Hope of Diabetics, Difficult and

Costly to Produce." With the initial cost of insulin treatment estimated at about $2 per day—more than half the typical daily earnings of an unskilled laborer back then, according to the U.S. Census—sales should have been topping a million dollars *per day* if all the estimated 550,000 diabetics in the country were buying it. But that was the amount that Lilly earned in its entire first year of selling the stuff.

Still, ramping up production and bringing down costs to get insulin to most of those who needed it was a relatively straightforward proposition in the boom years of the Roaring Twenties. Other problems, however, would not be so easily solved; indeed, they would only get worse for decades to come. Diabetes, it turned out, had more tricks up its sleeves than a vaudeville magician. After 3,500 years of playing humanity for a siphon, the evil flow of honey-sweet urine was just getting started.

CHAPTER 2

Two Steps Back

Deaths Continue Rising Despite Insulin and Pills,
1923–1975

C HARLIE BEST HAD SOME explaining to do. The co-discoverer of insulin had been invited to address the 127th annual meeting of the Medical Society of the State of New York, held on April 5, 1933, at the Waldorf-Astoria. His remarks were broadcast to New Yorkers on radio station WOR. In his speech on "The Story of Insulin," Dr. Best proudly told how he, Banting, Macleod, and Collip had discovered it over a decade earlier. Since then, he estimated, about 1 million people across the globe owed their lives to the discovery. Without insulin, he said, "These 1 million diabetics would have been condemned to death."

But there was a mystery to explain. Back in 1923, as previously noted, the death rate from diabetes in New York City was 22.9 per 100,000 residents. Now, with a treatment proved to quickly drop the blood-sugar rate down to normal, surely the diabetic death rate should have plummeted just as quickly. But instead, the death rate due to diabetes did something seriously strange: *it went up.* By 1926, it reached 25 per 100,000 residents of New York City. And it continued to rise every year thereafter, reaching 29 deaths due to diabetes per 100,000 New

Yorkers in 1932, a 26 percent increase over the 1923 rate. The conundrum was so puzzling that articles appeared in the *New York Times* with headlines like "Toll of Diabetes Is Rising Rapidly" and "Diabetes Mortality Up 58% in 30 Years." Some took the rise to mean that insulin, far from being a cure, was not even an effective treatment. There were even some doctors who refused to prescribe it.

Dr. Best had a simple explanation: the increase, he said, was due to the fact that Americans were living longer overall, and becoming increasingly likely to reach old age, when diabetes (at least the kind we now call type 2) is more likely to strike. There was some truth to this: the average life expectancy of New York City residents had in fact jumped from about 40 in the 1880s to about 55 by the middle of the 1920s. The historic increase in overall life expectancy was credited, in great measure, to improvements in sanitation and hygiene, and to the implementation of vaccines against infectious diseases. Once-feared diseases that had filled cemeteries with the pathetic graves of infants and children—from yellow fever and typhus to cholera, bubonic plague, and diphtheria—were now all but wiped out, at least in cities like New York. In Best's view, the increase in diabetes was simply a mathematical necessity, since whoever didn't die at a younger age would eventually have to die at an older age, of something else. It was thus left to the ravages of aging—not only diabetes, but also heart disease and cancer—to claim the lives of those who had been spared in youth. All things being equal, in other words, deaths due to diabetes couldn't help but go up as other causes of death went down.

But all things were not equal. One factor that Dr. Best had failed to mention was the ever-expanding waistline of the average New Yorker. According to the Statistical Bulletin of the Metropolitan Life Insurance Company released in June of 1929, "It is our best judgment that diabetes is on the increase, in spite of the use of insulin, because of the dietary excesses practiced by the American people." Four years later, a study conducted by Godias J. Drolet, statistician for the New York Tuberculosis and Health Association, found another striking trend: women, whose risk of death due to diabetes had been more or less equal to men's at the turn of the century, now had double the risk that men had. "In my opinion," Mr. Drolet said, "this increase among women is probably due to the noticeable release from physical labor and home drudgery, lightened by the so-called 'machine age' that the so-called modern woman of America enjoys. Diabetes is possibly a concomitant of reduced physical exercise—throwing a greater load on the internal organs."

But all of these explanations for the rise of diabetes—increasing age, increasing weight, and decreasing exercise—ignored one big thing: insulin. Even if growing numbers were becoming susceptible to diabetes, shouldn't insulin prevent them from dying from it? Remember, the German scientist Oskar Minkowski had proved back in 1889 that a dog without a pancreas developed diabetes, and Best and Banting had proved in 1922 that insulin was the magic ingredient in the pancreas that reversed the condition. Why should so many diabetics still be dying if the substance that their body lacked was being supplied to them with a simple daily injection?

Why, in other words, did 56-year-old Russell Foote, of 310 West 97th Street, die of diabetes on November 5, 1924, according to an obituary in the *New York Times,* at a time when insulin had become widely available in New York City? Why, after nearly 15 years of struggling with the disease, had he become so desperate two months earlier that he had cut his own throat "to end his misery"—at the very time when Best and Banting's great discovery offered relief? And why, after being taken to the Knickerbocker Hospital, where his gash had healed, and where he surely would have been given insulin if he hadn't obtained it on his own previously, did he nevertheless "die from the disease from which he suffered"?

Why didn't insulin save Russell Foote?

THE DISCOVERY OF INSULIN RESISTANCE

Doctors noticed something odd about insulin from the moment it escaped the confines of Best and Banting's laboratory in Toronto and made its way into their little black bags: the dose needed to help any given person varied wildly. Physicians and pharmacists were used to following standard dosing regimens for drugs like aspirin, ether, chloroform, or cocaine. Indeed, even today, there isn't an over-the-counter drug in our medicine chests without standard doses listed on the label. Of course, we logically expect that a larger person might need a larger dose of a given drug to achieve the same benefit, which is why a few shots of Jack Daniel's will have far less of an effect on a 220-pound football player than on a 110-pound cheerleader. We also know that the body can develop a tolerance for certain drugs, which is why that same cheerleader could drink the football player under the table if she's an alcoholic and he had previously been a teetotaler. But insulin followed none of these logical patterns. Some diabetics needed only 20 units of insulin per day to prevent them from spilling sugar into their urine; others required 200 units per day or more; and cases were described in which even 1,700 units of insulin were necessary to save a diabetic's life.

The first attempt to make sense of the mystery came in 1931, when a Viennese researcher, Professor Wilhelm Falta, published a paper in German describing what he considered to be two types of diabetes: *insularer*, or insulin-sensitive, and *insulinresistenter*, or insulin-resistant. Five years later, Falta's observations were confirmed and extended by Dr. Harold P. Himsworth, a brilliant young physician who had grown up in a working-class background, left school at 16 to take a job in a woolen mill, and gained entry to London's prestigious University College after studying nights for his entrance exam, thereby becoming the first in his family to leave Yorkshire county and the first to attend a university. After publishing five studies before the age of 30, Himsworth set out to develop a test that would clearly distinguish between the two types of diabetes.

To do so, Dr. Himsworth invited a number of patients to spend one evening and the following morning at University College's hospital, where he was by now the deputy director of the medical unit. After dinner, Dr. Himsworth allowed his patients no snacks and gave them no more insulin. The following morning he had them drink a dose of glucose dissolved in water flavored with citric acid and essence of lemon, and then gave them insulin intravenously. To standardize the amount of glucose and insulin based on the patients' height and weight, he gave 30 grams of glucose and five units of insulin for every square meter of their body surface. He then tested their blood-sugar level regularly for the next 90 minutes.

Writing in the January 18, 1936, edition of *The Lancet,* a prominent British medical journal, Himsworth described what he found: "The work had not proceeded far before it became clear that by means of this test diabetics can be differentiated into two types: those in whom the injected insulin produces an immediate suppression of the hyperglycemia [high blood-sugar level] which normally follows ingestion of glucose alone; and those in whom the insulin has little or no effect in suppressing this hyperglycemia." For instance, the first patient he tested, a 60-year-old woman, woke up with a blood-sugar level of 208 milligrams, far above the normal level of under 100. He gave her 7.3 units of insulin and 43.8 grams of glucose. Fifty minutes later, her blood-sugar level had jumped to 300; after another 40 minutes, when the test was over, her blood-sugar level had hit 360. In fact, hers was the reaction one would expect in a diabetic given *no insulin at all.* Himsworth thus labeled the woman, and diabetics like her, as "insulin-insensitive."

The results on the second patient, a 21-year-old woman, were dramatically different. She began with a blood-sugar level that was higher than the older woman's had been, 244. But 30 minutes after receiving seven units of insulin and 41 grams of glucose, her blood sugar *fell* to less than 180. It then began inching back up, returning to just under 240, before declining again, to 230, by the end of the 90-minute test. Himsworth labeled her, and patients like her, as "insulin-sensitive."

This was not just a matter of patients needing slightly more or less of the remedy that Best and Banting had discovered. Rather, these were really two different diseases, both of which resulted in high blood-sugar levels but only one of which could be easily treated with insulin. As Himsworth put it, "In the insulin-insensitive diabetic, insulin is unable to exert its characteristic action . . . Even if the insulin-insensitive patient possessed a normal supply of pancreatic insulin, such insulin would be unable to act efficiently and the patient would be diabetic."

He offered some tentative, broad observations on the two types of diabetes. "A general relationship appears to exist," he wrote, "between the type of onset of the disease and the type of diabetes. The onset in insulin-sensitive patients is as a rule acute; the onset in insulin-insensitive patients is insidious . . . . The insulin-insensitive type is more common in but not confined to the elderly, whilst the insulin-sensitive type is commoner in the young." He also reported that insulin-sensitive patients could eat a relatively normal amount of carbohydrate without spilling sugar into their urine (so long as they took their insulin), whereas people insensitive to insulin tended to spill sugar after only a modest increase in carbohydrate, even when they took insulin as prescribed.

What could explain the ineffectiveness of insulin in so many diabetics? It wasn't that the treatment was entirely ineffective, but that it required dramatically higher doses, on average, for those in whom diabetes had developed slowly, when they were older and overweight. Most researchers came to believe that there was some substance in such people's bodies that was blocking or resisting the insulin's normal action; these doctors called the condition "insulin resistance."

Himsworth took the opposite perspective: it wasn't something these patients *had* that was causing their trouble, but rather something they *lacked:* a sensitizing agent that makes insulin effective. Diabetics who responded to insulin had this sensitizing factor, he theorized, just as non-diabetics did. In Himsworth's view, then, the real problem for "insulin-insensitive" patients, as he called them, was not the lack of *insulin,* but the lack of *an unknown sensitizing factor.*

With no one able to say for certain what these unknown substances might be, "insulin resistance" became the standard term to describe the problem. Whatever the explanation, however, Himsworth had made a monumental discovery: diabetes is not a single disease. While Minkowski had proved 47 years earlier that an animal without a pancreas always develops diabetes, Himsworth had proved that supplying the insulin that is secreted by a healthy pancreas does not necessarily relieve the disease's symptoms. Far from being a cure, insulin, at least in the modest amounts normally supplied by the pancreas, was not even an effective treatment for those diabetics who were strangely insensitive to it.

And so the death rate from diabetes continued its relentless rise: from 29 per 100,000 New York City residents back in 1932, to 36.2 in January of 1936, to 38.8 for the full year of 1939. By then, the distinction between the two types was clear enough in the minds of some doctors that they thought they could explain away why so many "insulin-insensitive" patients were filling their offices.

Or, as Professor L. H. Newburgh of the University of Michigan told the Manitoba Medical Association in Winnipeg, half of all people diagnosed with diabetes are really "just gluttons, only they won't admit it. They're not diabetics at all, they're just fatties."

THE DISCOVERY OF COMPLICATIONS

Even for the younger, thinner diabetics for whom insulin easily lowered blood-sugar levels, it soon became apparent that it didn't protect them from developing all sorts of other ailments. Although microscopic damage to the kidneys had been observed in older diabetics as early as 1935, it took until 1951 for two doctors at Elliott Joslin's clinic in Boston, along with a Harvard medical student, to report on similar damage to the kidneys in young, thin diabetics. The Joslin team reviewed their clinic's records of 247 cases of long-standing diabetes in young people. The good news, of course, was that there were any such cases; before insulin, youthful diabetics simply did not survive long. The bad news, however, was that something was going terribly wrong with their kidneys, eyes, and blood vessels. As the Joslin team wrote: "Those patients who formerly died early in life of coma or acute infections are now avoiding or surviving these perils through the judicious use of insulin and antibiotics, only to succumb several years later to complications reflecting degenerative vascular disease."

Of the 247 long-standing cases, they found 62 patients, or 25 percent, with damage to their kidneys. All 62 of these patients had been spilling protein into their urine, a sign that the vessels in their kidneys had become leaky. High blood pressure was seen in 41 of the 62; bleeding of the tiny blood vessels in the eyes, called retinitis, occurred in 55; buildup of plaque within the arteries could be seen, via X-ray, in 47 of them. The longer the patients had diabetes, the Joslin team noted, the greater their chances of developing these dangerous complications. Just how dangerous was underscored by their review of 135 cases in which the patients had died between 1944 and 1950: 72 of them, or more than half, had evidence of kidney damage when examined on autopsy.

Amidst the gloom, however, the Joslin researchers emphasized that diabetics had the power to greatly reduce their risk of developing these complications by carefully following the regimen of diet and testing recommended by the Joslin clinic. The clinic urged diabetics to always weigh their food to estimate the precise amount of calories and carbohydrates; to test their urine for sugar every day; and to have regular physical exams and laboratory tests conducted by a physician. Out of all 247 cases they reviewed, not one diagnosis of kidney damage was made in those patients who had maintained "excellent control"—testing their urine more than once a day and adjusting their insulin dosage based on whether or not they were spilling sugar, weighing their food at least 80 percent of the time, undergoing annual examinations, and never once falling into a coma caused by a severely high blood-sugar level.

On the other hand, among the 62 patients with kidney damage, none had exercised better than "fair control"—meaning that they saw their doctors only once every two years, tested their urine only once or twice a week, and made only a half-hearted effort to follow their diet. Even those with "fair" control, however, had to have "rarely if ever indulged in gross dietary indiscretions," according to the Joslin team.

Not surprisingly, the record for those with "poor control" was worst of all. These patients had suffered coma from high sugar levels once or more; had sometimes taken their insulin irregularly; had tested their urine infrequently at best; had never weighed their foods; and had only rarely seen a doctor. Of the 62 patients with kidney disease, the Joslin team found, 80 percent fell into the "poor control" group. "Our data afford what we regard as convincing evidence," they concluded, "that careful, continuous control of diabetes does prevent or delay the onset of [kidney] complications among young diabetic patients."

The truth, however, was that many doctors had neither the time nor the training to provide the kind of intensive oversight of diabetes advocated by the Joslin Clinic. Complicated calculations had to be done to develop a precise diet for each patient based on his or her caloric needs. Patients then had to learn how to weigh all their foods and to base their insulin doses on whether or not they were spilling sugar into their urine. It was all too much for most doctors, and for most patients.

And it wasn't just the overworked family doctors who resisted the Joslin approach as impractical. Since the turn of the century, Elliott Joslin and his clinic had been synonymous with careful, continuous monitoring—what became known as "tight" control—of diabetics' diets and daily regimens. By the World War II era, it was not hard to form a caricature of Joslin as the crusty New Englander who simply couldn't lighten up and adjust to the freedom that insulin should have permitted.

Still, it is surprising that among those most avowedly hostile to Joslin's strict approach were some of the early leaders of the American Diabetes Association. In fact, at the very first annual meeting of the ADA, on June 1, 1941, the organization's second president, Dr. Herman O. Mosenthal, took the stage to directly challenge Joslin's approach. Having a high blood-sugar level, Mosenthal insisted, was not necessarily bad for diabetics. So long as they were not spilling sugar into their urine, he said, "A high blood sugar . . . is in all probability of no significance."

Even more outspoken against Joslin's hard line was Dr. Edward Tolstoi, one of the original founders of the ADA and a professor of medicine at Cornell University. He recommended giving diabetics only enough insulin to keep them feeling well, no matter what tests of their blood or urine might show. Rejecting Joslin's view that high sugar levels should never be seen in either the blood or the urine, Tolstoi wrote in 1948:

> Since the evidence that these are damaging is not substantiated by facts, but is only an impression, probably carried over from the pre-insulin era, we cannot see what is gained by straining one's effort to maintain the diabetic patient sugar free, except that the patient's day is either made or ruined, depending on what his specimen showed. He becomes a worrier. He feels he is different, and has a code of do's and don'ts, which do not help him psychologically. On the contrary, both [my] adult and juvenile diabetics lead normal lives, eat a generous diet—not weighed—have few rules—one of which is never to omit insulin—and I have convinced myself, and them, after a decade of observation from clinical and experimental studies, that as long as they feel well, are not hungry, thirsty, maintain their weight, and do not void frequently or much, their diabetes is well controlled.

As the experts continued their debates, diabetics continued dying at ever-rising rates. By 1947, despite the sugar rationing of the war years, and with the postwar baby boom adding 170,469 tiny new residents that year alone, New York City's death rate due to diabetes hit a new high, 44.4 per 100,000 people. That was almost *double* the 1923 rate and a staggering 31-fold increase over the Civil War rate. Like the rise of a backwater politician to the presidency, an obscure disease that had barely registered on the charts was now the sixth leading cause of death.

A LONGER-ACTING INSULIN

Trout sperm. This unlikeliest of substances proved to be the first in a long line of substances meant to replace or improve upon insulin. After all, maybe the secret to saving diabetics' lives—maybe even the secret to preventing people from becoming diabetic in the first place—could be found not in lecturing them to eat less or to test their urine more, but in a drug that succeeded where insulin had failed. That's where trout sperm came in.

Until 1936, the insulin sold to diabetics had been purified so well that it worked much faster than the original, impure insulin that Drs. Banting and Best had first extracted from cows back in 1921, but it acted for only a few hours at a time to lower blood-sugar levels. The result was not only the inconvenience of having to take three or four injections per day, but the danger of having sugar levels drop so fast and so low that the diabetic might pass out and even die.

Then a researcher at the Nordisk Insulin Laboratory in Copenhagen, Hans Hagedorn, had an idea: perhaps it was the very *impurities* in Banting and Best's original version that prevented their insulin from working quickly and kept it working longer. Perhaps, Hagedorn reasoned, adding a protein to the insulin would achieve the same moderating effect without causing the allergic reactions seen with Banting and Best's impurities. But where could he find a good source of soluble protein?

Hagedorn tested different sources before settling on, of all things, trout sperm. The protein in it, called protamine, did the trick when mixed with otherwise pure insulin. Soon after, a Toronto researcher thought to add zinc to the mixture, which made the insulin act even more slowly. By September of 1936, when Elliott Joslin was invited to speak at a gathering to celebrate Harvard Medical School's 300th anniversary, he stated that diabetics could now take a single shot of the new protamine zinc insulin once every other day. The new formulation, he said, would "promote the taking of insulin by more diabetics than ever before and thus prolong and maintain in comfort many diabetic lives." (It is worth noting that in its report on the speech, the *New York Times* misidentified protamine as "a chemical," not an extract of trout sperm.)

Whether the new, longer-acting insulin would indeed prolong lives was soon brought into question by a study presented in Denver at the June 1937 meeting of the American Association for the Advancement of Science. Dr. Eaton M. McKay and Richard H. Barnes, researchers from the Scripps Metabolic Institute of La Jolla, California, reported on how they had tried to reproduce in animals an effect that had been observed in humans: the unfortunate tendency of older, overweight diabetics to gain even more weight when given high enough doses of insulin to combat their insensitivity to it. When McKay and Barnes gave regular insulin to white rats, they did not gain weight. But when they gave them protamine zinc insulin, the rats "got so obese, like white puff balls, that they had difficulty rolling over."

THE FIRST PILL

With so many problems besetting the use of insulin—not least of which was the fear and loathing most people felt toward hypodermic needles—researchers began searching for an alternative that could be taken by mouth. As early as 1926, researchers in Minkowski's laboratory in Breslau reported that they had isolated the active ingredient in the herb *Galega officinalis* (popularly known as French lilac or goat's rue) responsible for its use as a diabetic folk remedy. At first it looked like they might have stumbled upon something as useful as willow tree bark, from which salicylic acid had been isolated and chemically manipulated into aspirin. The Breslau group successfully isolated the compound guanidine, which they then manipulated into a derivative they called synthalin, as in "synthetic insulin."

Synthalin was not a replacement for insulin, but merely prevented the liver from releasing its stores of glucose, as it normally does between meals. They hoped it would be a useful treatment for older, heavier diabetics whose pancreases produced insulin. Unfortunately, it soon became apparent that synthalin caused toxic side effects by interfering with the liver's functioning. Despite a flurry of papers from groups in Europe and the United States quickly confirming synthalin's ability to lower sugar levels, the toxic side effects were also confirmed, and synthalin's brief flirtation with the European market ended.

The first true breakthrough in the search for a pill grew out of the privations of World War II. In the spring of 1942, in the French Mediterranean city of Montpellier, people were getting so desperate for food that they began eating rotting or contaminated meat and seafood. The many resulting cases of typhoid fever were treated by Dr. Marcel Janbon of the Montpellier Medical School with one of the miraculous new sulfa drugs that had revolutionized the treatment of bacterial infections. But the sulfa drug he chose, an experimental one known simply as 2254 RP, turned out to cause some severe side effects of its own: convulsions and coma.

Dr. Janbon asked a physiologist at the medical school, Auguste Loubatières, to look into the matter. Loubatières had been studying protamine zinc insulin, and he suspected that the side effects caused by 2254 RP were the result of severely low sugar levels, the kind that could be caused by taking too much insulin. On June 13, 1942, Loubatières gave 2254 RP to a dog, and sure enough, tests showed that the dog's blood-sugar level dropped dramatically.

Loubatières and Janbon kept up their experiments throughout the war, eventually concluding that the drug worked by spurring what they called a "lazy" pancreas into producing more insulin. But once the Nazis had rolled into Montpellier and learned of the work, Germany's pharmaceutical giants sought to exploit the results with other sulfa drugs. A Dresden firm, Chemische Fabrik von Heyden, identified one called BZ 55, or carbutamide. Its research efforts collapsed with the ruins of the Third Reich, when Dresden became part of East Germany. It took until 1952 for a sample of carbutamide to be smuggled across the Iron Curtain into West Germany, where it was tested and brought onto the German market in 1956. Further testing in the United States revealed rare but fatal side effects that resulted in its discontinuation.

But in 1957, another sugar-lowering sulfa drug (the technical name for such a drug is sulfonylurea) was brought onto the U.S. market by an American firm, the Upjohn Company. The result was a pharmaceutical juggernaut that would transform the very definition of diabetes.

MAKING LEMONADE

Orinase, as the drug was called, offered a tricky marketing challenge for Upjohn. The company had brought in top researchers from across the United States, including some from the Joslin Clinic, to test it on over 5,000 patients. What they found would have disappointed a less ambitious drug company: Orinase didn't work for most people with diabetes who already took insulin; all it did was stimulate a functioning pancreas to work a little harder. Young, thin people with diabetes didn't have a properly functioning pancreas, and many of the older, heavier people with diabetes who had to take large doses of insulin to overcome their resistance needed more than Orinase could coax out of their pancreas.

The people in whom Orinase worked best, in fact, were precisely those in whom insulin injections had traditionally been considered unnecessary: older diabetics with a mild, early form of the disease. Still,

36

with no signs of serious side effects, and on the strength of an extraordinary 10,580-page application document, Orinase won FDA approval.

Taking what some would consider a lemon, the Upjohn marketing department began selling lemonade. As described in exquisite detail by Harvard physician-historian Jeremy A. Greene in *Prescribing by Numbers: Drugs and the Definitions of Diseases* (Johns Hopkins University Press, 2007), Upjohn succeeded in convincing doctors that these mild cases, often undiagnosed, needed to be found and treated. The odd thing was that people with so-called "hidden" diabetes, or "pre-diabetes," had none of the symptoms that had defined the disease for millennia. A promotional film made by Upjohn and described in Dr. Greene's book attacked the problem head-on, asking "how we convince people who do not feel sick, do not feel that they are patients," to begin taking a drug for a disease they never knew they had.

It's not that Upjohn was creating a disease category out of thin air: most of these early diabetics would, in fact, progress to full diabetes over time, and they did have increased risks for developing the long-term complications associated with the disease. And while there was no clear evidence, the logical assumption that lowering sugar levels should lower their long-term risks of complications was hard to refute. Maybe the drug would even prevent their diabetes from becoming more severe. And so in 1958, Orinase was being taken by 320,000 of the estimated 1.5 million people diagnosed with diabetes in the United States.

Close on the heels of Orinase, another sulfonylurea hit the U.S. market, Diabinese, launched by Pfizer & Co. with an unprecedented 24-page advertising insert in the *Journal of the American Medical Association*. Almost simultaneously, a third drug came out, not from pharmaceutical giants like Upjohn or Pfizer but from a little-known firm with scant experience in selling drugs, U.S. Vitamin Corporation. Seymour L. Shapiro, a chemist at the company who had diabetes himself, had gone back to the old drug synthalin to chemically tinker with it in hopes of eliminating the toxic side effects. He came up with one called phenformin, later sold under the trade name DBI. It seemed to have no side effects beyond causing nausea or diarrhea in some people, which could usually be relieved by lowering the dose. Like Orinase and Diabinese, it worked only in the older, heavier diabetics. (Such patients were now said to have "adult-onset" diabetes, as opposed to "juvenile" diabetes.) But unlike its competitors, which usually caused weight gain, phenformin often led to weight loss. It even reduced cholesterol levels!

By the time the conservative crew cuts of the Eisenhower era had given way to mop-tops and go-go boots, the defeat of diabetes appeared well in hand. Doctors were happy to have so many choices for treating their patients; patients were happy to have pills rather than being stuck between a rock (insulin syringes) and a hard place (draconian diets); and the drug companies were happy to be making money while doing good. Everything was beautiful.

Or so it seemed. Despite the apparent progress, the number of diabetics was still going up, along with the severe complications. From an estimate of 2 million people with diabetes in 1960, or 9 out of every 1,000 people, the number of known cases in the United States grew to about 2.3 million in 1965, or 12.2 per thousand. By the end of the turbulent decade, diabetes was the country's leading cause of kidney failure, the leading cause of adult-onset blindness, and the leading cause of amputation.

And then something called the UGDP hit the fan.

AN INCONVENIENT STUDY

On May 20, 1970, the results of the largest diabetes study ever conducted were leaked, unofficially and before being published in a medical journal or presented at a medical meeting, by the Dow Jones newswire. The next morning, a longer article about the study appeared in the *Washington Post*. The University Group Diabetes Program, or UGDP, had been started ten years earlier to do what no drug company had: track the long-term death rates of diabetics on pills, insulin, or diet alone. The findings were shocking: during eight years of follow-up, 26 out of 204 patients on Orinase, or 12.7 percent, had died of heart disease, compared to just 10 of 205 patients (4.9 percent) who had been given a placebo. People taking insulin, on the other hand, had a risk of death due to heart disease that was no higher than people managing their diabetes by diet alone. The results were significant enough that the leaders of the UGDP had decided to stop the Orinase portion of the study early.

The reaction was swift and cataclysmic. As Dr. Greene puts it in *Prescribing by Numbers,* "All hell broke loose." An estimated 800,000 Americans, he notes, "were taking Orinase every day for mild (asymptomatic) diabetes, largely on the premise that the pill reduced their long-term risk for diabetic complications and heart disease." Leading diabetes specialists at Joslin and the ADA expressed outrage—not at drug manufacturers but at the press, for daring to report the study before it had been presented at the annual meeting of the ADA in June, and at the academics who had designed it, whom they accused of sloppy statistical work. The medical equivalent of a soap opera played itself out before a perplexed and whipsawed public.

On June 8, the FDA sent a letter to physicians noting that sulfonylureas "could no longer be given simply on the ground that they might help and could do no harm." A week later, the ADA responded by saying it saw no need to abandon the use of oral medications. The American Medical Association, on the other hand, supported the FDA's cautious view. That fall, a group of 34 leading diabetes specialists led by Dr. Robert F. Bradley, medical director of the Joslin Clinic, held a press conference known as the "Boston Tea Party," in which they renounced the views of the FDA and AMA. Dr. Bradley went so far as to call the UGDP study "worthless."

In October 1970, the ADA reversed itself, saying it now agreed with the AMA and the FDA that Orinase should be taken only by adult-onset diabetics in whom diet has failed and insulin is unacceptable or impractical. In December, Bradley and his Boston Tea Party, now going under the more dignified name of "Committee for the Care of the Diabetic," deplored the warning letter the FDA had mailed out to physicians, saying it had "damaged the welfare of a million diabetic patients" and was guilty of "unprecedented interference with the practice of medicine."

In May of 1971, phenformin was dragged into the debate. The UGDP had studied it, too, and only now were the results available: 26 out of 204 patients on phenformin died of heart disease (12.7 percent), compared to only 2 of 64 patients given a placebo (3.1 percent). That same month, the FDA announced its intention to require all pills sold for diabetes to include a special warning on the label about the apparent increased risk of death due to heart disease. Faced with a harsh response from Bradley and his growing group of followers, who filed a lawsuit to prevent the action, the agency reconsidered.

By 1975, with an astonishing 1.5 million people now taking pills for diabetes, the FDA again proposed to require stern warnings on the labels, saying the drugs "may be associated with increased cardiovascular mortality as compared to treatment with diet alone or diet plus insulin." An investigator with the National Institutes of Health, brought in to help review the statistical evidence for or against the pills, estimated that they were causing 10,000 to 15,000 deaths per year.

Yet that spring, the chief executive officer of the AMA permitted Upjohn to use a letter he wrote minimizing the risks of the drugs, even though the AMA's journal had published a study confirming those risks. At a hearing in August, one of the UGDP investigators was charged with having been on the payroll of a competitor of Upjohn, and the FDA was warned it would "be on mighty thin ice" if it tried going ahead with the proposed warning on the label.

Why were the very specialists who should have been defending the health and welfare of diabetics instead defending the drugs? Because the drugs really did lower blood-sugar levels, and the patients really did like them. It is impossible to exaggerate how resistant most grown men and women, then as now, are to following strict diets, or how much they dislike the prospect of taking shots. And there was some evidence that by lowering sugar levels, the pills did lower the risk of damage to the eyes and other organs, if not the heart.

On a deeper level, though, the dynamics between those defending and those attacking the pills were ultimately determined by the kind of evidence, and the kind of government, they believed in. On one side of the UGDP battlefield stood those who swore by the results of large studies and believed that government should protect and defend the people's well-being. Among the defenders of this view were the FDA, academics, and consumer-protection groups like the Health Research Group formed by Ralph Nader's Public Citizen. On the other side stood practitioners (urged on by self-interested manufacturers) who placed their faith in their own hands-on experience with patients, and whose libertarian politics deemed the FDA and other would-be regulators as interlopers.

Far from discouraged, indeed, the spirit of diabetes specialists grew ever more optimistic in the 1970s as a wave of new treatments became available. A new, more liberal diet was approved by the ADA, encouraging diabetics to eat the same kind of low-fat, high-carbohydrate diet that was being urged upon all Americans. The chemical structure of insulin was fully synthesized, paving the way for industrial production without the need for pancreases from slaughtered cows and pigs. Lasers were studied as a tool for treating diabetics' eye disease. The first transplants of human pancreases were performed, soon followed by the first transplants of insulin-producing islet cells. So many exciting, high-tech developments were underway that it was said by some that diabetes would likely be cured within a decade.

REALITY CHECK

But late in 1975, a different, and decidedly darker, picture of diabetes in America came from the National Commission on Diabetes, a government-funded group that had been asked by Congress to take a cold, hard look at the disease and its treatment. Baseball legend Jackie Robinson had died of complications of the disease in 1972, at the age of 53, and cartoonist Walt Kelly, creator of "Pogo" (the "Doonesbury" of its day), had died of it in 1973 at the age of 60. The commission announced that diabetes was now responsible for more than 300,000 deaths per year in the United States, making it the third-leading cause of death, behind only heart disease and cancer.

In all, the number of people diagnosed with diabetes stood at 5 million, and another 5 million had the disease but didn't know it. Both these figures, for diagnosed and undiagnosed diabetes, were 250 percent above the figures cited in 1960. More than 50 years after the discovery of insulin, the commission told Congress, little progress had been made in treating the disease. Diabetics' risk of developing heart disease was double that of non-diabetics, their risk of going blind was 25 times higher, and their overall life expectancy was one-third shorter.

Were all the drugs and all the treatments of the modern American healthcare system incapable of improving and extending the lives of people with diabetes? Could it even be that they were only making things worse? It would take the next phase in the history of diabetes, the modern era of "tight control," for answers to finally come into focus.

CHAPTER 3

Try Harder

The Rise of Tight Control for Type 1: 1975 to Present Day

LEARNED ABOUT THE RISE of tight control the hard way. I lived through it.

My last supper as a non-diabetic was on Thanksgiving Day of 1975. I felt so nauseated and exhausted that day at my brother's home in Iowa, where I had hitchhiked for the holiday, that I barely made it to the dinner table. Thirty-four years later, I still remember the tiny forkful of stuffing that I brought to my mouth that evening, and the even tinier crumb of it that I forced myself to swallow. That was my Thanksgiving meal.

On the bus ride back to Beloit College, where I was in my freshman year, my mouth was so dry that I insisted to the driver that I absolutely had to get out at a rest stop to buy a soda. Returning to my seat as the bus pulled out, I drank the entire contents of the Coke in a single long gulp.

"You really must have been thirsty," someone sitting in front of me said.

When I opened my mouth to reply, my throat was so parched that I couldn't speak.

Still sick to my stomach the next day, I was sent by the school nurse to the local emergency room. Sitting there on a cold metal examination cubicle in a drafty hospital gown, waiting for a physician, I began to put things together. Since arriving at college a few months earlier, I'd been slowly but steadily losing weight, maybe 15 pounds. I was always thirsty and always peeing. And now here I was, vomiting like a geyser. This was no flu. This was something serious. It was cancer. I was dying.

When the curtain on the examination cubicle parted and the doctor pronounced the word *diabetes,* he might as well have said multiple sclerosis or the plague or cancer, for all it meant to me. Hey, I was an English major.

The next morning, the indoctrination began. First came the nurse, to explain how and when and where I would inject the insulin: once in the morning and once at night, in my thighs, biceps, or stomach. She gave me an orange to practice injecting. I was actually very lucky, she assured me; there were now plastic disposable needles being sold, so I wouldn't have to buy a glass syringe and boil it after every use.

Then came the dietitian. I would now eat on a schedule. It was all in the little booklet. For breakfast, at 8 A.M., I would have two pieces of bread or one cup of cereal with a piece of fruit, some protein—an egg, maybe, or a sausage, or some peanut butter—all washed down with a glass of milk. And I could have a pat of butter with that if I felt like it. See how easy? At 10:30 A.M., I'd have a snack: a slice of bread and another glass of milk. Or I could have cottage cheese or yogurt. I could even substitute a piece of fruit. It was really quite flexible. But not a candy bar. Or ice cream, cake, pie, juice, soda, or anything sweet. But coffee was fine, along with sugar-free Jell-O, lettuce, diet soda, and broccoli. Failure to comply could result in such complications as coma, blindness, amputation, kidney failure, impotence, and death.

That afternoon, the doctor who'd diagnosed me in the emergency room came by to see how I was doing. When I told him it all seemed kind of overwhelming, he gave me some advice to try to put all the rules into perspective: "If you used to have two scoops of ice cream, now you have one. If you used to have a slice of cake every night after dinner, now you have half a slice."

That was actually not the advice of a screwball. A legitimate school of thought in those days still held, as leading diabetes specialists had advocated since the 1940s, that diabetics should not fuss overly much about their disease, that they should just take their daily shot or two, follow a simple diet as well as they could, and get on with it. And so the gist of the message I got was that diabetes is no big deal. After all, a cure was right around the corner—surgeons had recently figured out how to transplant pancreases!

Happy to follow the "don't worry, be happy" line on diabetes care, I landed in the hospital three times in the next five years with life-threatening bouts of severe low blood-sugar levels, also known as hypoglycemia. Hypoglycemia is a dangerous condition in which one's sugar level falls too low for the brain to properly function. Usually it causes just mild symptoms—dizziness, confusion, anxiety, sweating, and jitteriness—which usually prompt the person to drink some juice, pop a glucose tab, or munch down on some Life Savers. But if the person doesn't notice the symptoms, or is sleeping, or for any other reason doesn't grab something sweet, then loss of consciousness can result, and even death.

I never tested my sugar level at home in those days, because no test strips were sold for self-testing. The best hope for avoiding hypoglycemia was to take the exact same amount of insulin, eat the exact same amount of carbohydrate, and do the exact same amount of exercise every day. Find a routine that works, and stick with it. Which I, being way too smart for anything so simple and effective, never did.

COOL TOOLS

And then one evening in the autumn of 1980, a friend who worked at the St. Louis chapter of the American Diabetes Association brought me something nifty: a little canister containing specially coated strips that would change color based on how high or low my sugar level was. All I had to do was prick my finger to get a drop of blood and place it on the strip. The problem was, my friend hadn't brought along one of the new, automatic, spring-loaded lancets that quickly and painlessly prick one's finger. So I found a sewing needle and began jabbing away. It was awful, but it worked. I got a drop of blood, blotted it onto the test strip, waited a minute, wiped it clean, and waited another minute.

The strip had turned deep blue. Checking the color against the ranges on the canister, I saw that my blood-sugar level was somewhere between 180 and 240.

"Pretty cool," my friend said.

"Yeah," I said. "Cool."

Without knowing what, if anything, I should do in response to a particular sugar level, it was just a parlor trick. But that knowledge would come. The first great tool of the tight-control movement had arrived. Soon, doctors and nurses would be teaching patients how to adjust their diet and insulin levels to maintain near-normal sugar levels.

The second great tool that heralded the rise of tight control was for use by doctors. Back in 1976, researchers had reported on a blood test that revealed the average level of sugar (or glucose, as the sugar in blood is known) over a three- or four-month period. The hemoglobin molecules in blood, studies showed, bond with glucose molecules depending on how much glucose is floating in the blood. These sugar-coated hemoglobin molecules are said to be "glycosylated." And because the average lifespan of hemoglobin molecules is about 120 days, checking for the percent of them that have been sugar-coated gives doctors a rough measure of how often, during those preceding 120 days, a person's sugars have been high. By the early 1980s, a consensus had emerged that this test, called the glycosylated hemoglobin A1C (or simply the "A1C" test), could tell doctors and patients how good a job they were doing, overall, at controlling their sugar level.

I first fell under the spell of the tight controllers in 1986, after moving to New York City and coming under the care of Zachary Bloomgarden, MD, a strong believer in the approach. Dr. Bloomgarden taught me to test my blood sugars not once or twice a day but five to eight times, keeping detailed written logs of the results and always striving to keep my sugars under 200. It became a game of math, motivation, and maturity.

Of course, tight control wasn't for everyone. I became friendly with another guy who had type 1 diabetes, lived in my neighborhood in Brooklyn and wrote regularly for *The New Yorker.* When I told him how often I tested my sugars and took tiny corrective doses of insulin in response, he looked at me as if I had gone nuts. "I'd rather die than live like that," he said. And then he did, some years later, of a severe hypoglycemic reaction from which he never awoke.

As a matter of pure science, however, the tight-control hypothesis remained precisely that: a hypothesis for which the evidence remained equivocal. It seemed sensible. To some, it seemed beyond dispute that getting sugar levels near to normal would reduce complications. But then, scientific progress is built on the graves of hypotheses that once seemed indisputable.

"The idea that some doctors thought they knew best was interesting but totally unfounded," said one of the leading researchers in the field, David M. Nathan, MD, professor of medicine at Harvard Medical School and director of the General Clinical Research Center and of the Diabetes Center at Massachusetts General Hospital. "Randomized trials are the only kind of experiments that can assess the magnitude of the benefits and the magnitude of the side effects for any therapy. Insights are great, theories are great, but when it comes down to implementing therapies with human beings who can suffer the benefits as well as the risks, there's no doubt you need to do randomized trials. Otherwise you might as well go on TV and advertise Extenz. It's hucksterism."

FROM THEORY TO GOSPEL

The tipping point for the tight-control hypothesis came on the morning of Sunday, June 13, 1993, when a standing-room-only audience crowded into the vast main ballroom of the Las Vegas Convention Center. The premier event of the annual ADA meeting that year was the scheduled announcement of the results of the Diabetes Control and Complications Trial, or DCCT, launched ten years earlier at 29 medical centers in the United States and Canada, eventually recruiting 1,441 people with type 1 diabetes, all of them under age 40 and free of serious complications at the outset.

Half the diabetics in the DCCT had been placed on conventional care, testing their sugars once a day, taking one or two daily insulin injections, and following dietary advice as best they could on their own. The other half were taught to test their sugars four to seven times a day and to take insulin three to five times daily based on how high or low their sugars were. Nurses, doctors, and dietitians kept in close contact with them, even having weekly telephone calls with each participant. A1C tests were conducted regularly to compare the two groups' average sugar levels. At the conclusion of the study, the researchers assessed the diabetics for signs of new or progressive complications, including eye disease, nerve damage, and evidence of kidney dysfunction.

Now, at last, they would report whether all the work and hardship of the patients and doctors involved in the DCCT had been worth it. As if any additional drama could be added, everyone in attendance at the meeting knew that the study had been cut short by a year, when the results had become clear enough that any further testing would be unethical to the half of patients receiving the less beneficial treatment. *But which half?*

No one awaited the results more eagerly than I, sitting in the front row of the cavernous auditorium. As a reporter for the *Medical Tribune*, which distributed articles to newspapers across the United States via the *New York Times* wire service, I had finagled myself an assignment to cover the meeting. I listened and typed notes on a laptop as one researcher after another took the podium to describe first the overall design of the study, then the details of how the patients were tested and instructed, then the statistical measures used to gauge the results, and finally, at long last, the results. And the researcher who presented them was—who else?—David M. Nathan, MD, the youngest member of the team of principal investigators who led the DCCT.

The doctors, reporters, and people with diabetes sitting in the audience knew, as I did, that a normal A1C, for people without diabetes, is under 6.0. They also knew that with poorly managed, out-of-control diabetes, an A1C can be 12.0 or higher. Now came the moment of truth, as Dr. Nathan reported the results of the DCCT. The tight-control group, he told us, had an average A1C of 7.2. The conventional-care group had an average A1C of 8.9—much higher. So the regimen had certainly succeeded in lowering average sugar levels. But what difference did that make for altering health outcomes? Compared to those who received conventional care, the people assigned to the tight-control group had:

- 76% less risk of developing initial signs of eye disease if they never had it before;

- 54% less risk of worsening eye disease if they had early signs of it at the beginning of the study;

- 39% less risk of spilling small amounts of protein in their urine, a sign of early kidney disease;

- 54% less risk of spilling higher amounts of protein;

- 60% less risk of developing neuropathy, a painful nerve disorder in the feet and hands.

There was just one catch, Dr. Nathan informed us: the tight-control group was about three times more likely to have severe hypoglycemic events, where their blood-sugar levels fell so low that they needed somebody's assistance. The short-term risk of bad lows, it seemed, was the unavoidable price to pay for reducing the long-term risks of blindness, kidney failure, and nerve damage.

The presentation ended with spontaneous applause, even cheering. The head of the National Institute of Diabetes and Digestive and Kidney Diseases (NIDDK), which had funded the study, compared the importance of the DCCT to the discovery of insulin. Although the study had involved only type 1 diabetics, the implication was that getting the sugar levels of type 2 as close to normal as possible would have similar benefits.

I found myself flushed with excitement. But as I began to pack up my computer, my sense of thrill became tinged with confusion, even anxiety. I felt myself sweating profusely. What was wrong? I opened my canister of Chemstrips BG, pulled out a strip, pricked my finger with a lancet, dabbed a drop of blood onto the strip, waited a minute, wiped the blood off the strip, and waited another minute. It was pale blue. My sugar level was somewhere around 40—far lower than normal, which is about 80, and low enough to make me feel mixed up, sweaty, and just plain awful. (It's really a rather nightmarish feeling, comparable to the freaked-out way you might feel if you had just been in a minor automobile accident.) I dug out some Life Savers from the bottom of my computer bag as it occurred to me that I was experiencing the very drawback to tight control that had been seen in the DCCT.

Out in the hallway, walking briskly toward the press room and its spread of refreshments, I passed a knot of attendees wearing large buttons that said, "We Told You So." They were the people from Joslin, unable to refrain from a little in-your-face celebrating of their late founder's faith in tight control having been finally vindicated.

But it was one thing to demonstrate the benefits of tight control in a study of type 1 diabetics, all of them young, motivated, otherwise healthy, and treated to the free care of leading endocrinologists and specially trained nurses and dietitians at the top academic medical centers in North America. It would be another thing entirely to find the same level of benefits, without an even greater risk of severe hypoglycemia, among type 1s in the real world, let alone type 2s, in whom no study of tight control had yet been conducted. Later that morning, after my own sugar level had stabilized, I tracked down Dr. Nathan to get his view of how the field might implement the DCCT's findings.

"Educating primary-care doctors in how to instruct their patients in intensive management of diabetes is probably not feasible," he told me. "It's too complicated."

Another leader of the study, William Tamborlane, MD, of Yale, told me, "There are tremendous burdens of this therapy day-to-day, and it's highly risky."

Yet almost overnight, tight control went from theory to gospel, and getting blood sugars as near to normal as possible, without going too low, became the first commandment of diabetes care.

GADGET FEVER

Spreading that gospel proved challenging. With fewer than 6,000 board-certified endocrinologists (the medical specialists who treat diabetes) in the entire United States, most of them clustered in major cities, the sheer logistics of communicating the new treatment strategy to so many people of all ages and personalities and economic and social backgrounds were daunting. Even as the number of nurses and dietitians specially trained in diabetes education grew, the expense and complexity of state-of-the-art care for type 1 grew faster.

Do the math: with test strips retailing between 75¢ and $1 each, and the tight-control regimen in the DCCT involving an average of six tests per day, that would be at least $4.50 per day per diabetic, or $1,642.50 per year, multiplied by 1.4 million if all the people in the United States then estimated to have type 1 immediately began following the new regimen, which would exceed *$2 billion a year*. Not counting doctors' visits, eye exams, insulin, or anything else.

As an early adopter, I didn't need convincing that tight control was worth the hassles. But I also knew that by carefully following my doctor's advice to keep my blood-sugar levels as close to normal as possible, I always lived on the edge, a cupcake away from a coma. Every day or two, I got a brief, mild low that left me feeling muddle-headed and cranky for half an hour. (It happened this afternoon as I was working on this chapter.) Not the end of the world, but a definite annoyance and productivity-killer.

And then there were the scary times. On Cape Cod for a two-week vacation in August of 2005, I went to sleep one night and almost never woke up. I had developed such severe hypoglycemia that my daughter, Annie, then all of nine years old, found me unresponsive and soaked in sweat in the morning. With my wife, Alice, in New Jersey for a couple of days to attend a meeting, Annie managed to dribble some grape soda into my mouth, followed by a few spoonfuls of Marshmallow Fluff. Fifteen minutes later, my blood sugar rising, I came to my senses enough to think, "Not again!"

It's easy to see, then, why people with type 1 began buying into yet another tool to help control their diabetes. Priced at over $5,000 each, with an additional expense of hundreds more per month in supplies, external insulin pumps were pitched as a way to make frequent, small changes in insulin dosing more feasible, to eliminate the unpredictable swings in sugar levels caused by the action of long-acting insulins, and to permit diabetics greater freedom in deciding when and how much to eat. For the well-educated and well-to-do who could best afford them, they also conveyed an undeniable aura of high-tech cachet. Inserted less than an inch deep with a spring-loaded injector into a diabetic's abdomen or backside, a cannula was then attached to a computerized pumping device to release insulin as programmed. Although primitive insulin pumps had been around since the late 1970s (thanks in large part to Dr. Tamborlane's pioneering research at Yale), they gained new currency from the DCCT's inclusion of "pumpers" in the tight-control group, and from their growing computer power.

I finally decided to go on a pump in 1999, after my insurance company agreed to pay much of the cost. On balance, I found it made life easier by allowing me to make minor adjustments in my insulin rates on the fly, but resulted in little change to my A1C numbers. And my lows remained every bit as common as my highs. Essentially, it was just another way, albeit incrementally better, to get the same old insulin I'd always used. And while friends and family often assumed that the pump worked like an artificial pancreas, giving me only as much insulin as I needed, in fact it was as dumb as a brick, following only the instructions I gave it. Like jet packs, hover cars, and daily flights to the moon, the artificial pancreas remained nothing more than an alluring fantasy at the turn of the millennium.

Then, on August 10, 2005, the FDA finally approved the next critical step toward an artificial pancreas: an implantable glucose sensor for continuously measuring sugar levels. Although few if any insurance companies were willing to cover the costs of such sensors, I managed to convince my editor at the *New York Times,* for which I wrote freelance articles on health and science, to assign me to test one of the approved devices and write about my experience.

TEST DRIVE

On Monday, June 12, 2006, I took the train down to Washington to be hooked up to one while the annual meeting of the ADA was in town. The device, made by Medtronic MiniMed, was called the Paradigm Real-Time, a combination insulin pump and continuous glucose sensor. The sensor didn't actually control the pump; it only gave readouts of glucose levels, updated every five minutes, which presumably would allow a diabetic to make quicker, better decisions. Still, anything that would allow me to see a low coming, and pop a few Life Savers to prevent it, seemed like a dream come true.

The big problem with developing a workable, reliable sensor was in finding something that could be placed inside the human body for days at a time that wouldn't cause a blood clot, wouldn't get coated by scar tissue, and was, by the way, reliably accurate. For years bio-engineers had tested devices placed directly in the bloodstream, eventually concluding it was too challenging and dangerous to be practical.

Then they began tinkering to see if they could measure the sugar level in the interstitial fluid, the juice floating between fat cells right under the skin. Sure enough, they developed a coated metal tip that measured the electrical conductivity of the interstitial fluid by sending out imperceptibly tiny electrical charges. As luck would have it, the conductivity turned out to be directly proportional to how much glucose was floating around in the juice.

Medtronic sent three of its senior medical personnel, including two of its top physician-researchers, to train me in how to use their sensor. Like the pump, I learned, the sensor requires injecting a tiny catheter (less than an inch long) into the midsection of the body, and changing it every three days to avoid infection. Even with the help of a roomful of experts, however, I found the insertion process tricky. They wanted me to place it above the hip or in the buttocks, which made reaching it awkward. And once that was done, I had to click onto the end of the sensor a transmitter that wirelessly sends data to the pump, which stores and reads out the information. Sound confusing? It was.

When everything was in, I had two catheters and the transmitter all taped to my body, plus the pump hanging on my belt. Kind of weird, but kind of cool, in a sci-fi way, and I remained thrilled at the prospect of seeing my first glucose reading.

Then the waiting began. The sensor needed three hours to settle in before it could begin transmitting data. By late afternoon, when it was supposed to start, I got an error message instead. When I tried to recalibrate it a half hour later, it still wasn't working right, so I had to remove it and inject a second one. It was after 9 P.M. before the second one finally began working.

At first, I was transfixed by the numbers as they were updated every five minutes. That night, however, the sensor kept beeping me awake, nearly every hour, warning that my glucose level was too high.

I kept following the recommendations of the embedded calculator, taking only very small amounts of insulin to bring my sugar level down. But by morning I was still high, so I followed my own usual guesstimate and took much more.

Two hours later, while attending a session at the ADA meeting, in which four experts talked about the new sensors, I heard mine beep again, this time warning me that my glucose level was plummeting. I quickly drank a juice box, and within minutes my numbers started leveling off. I had avoided my first low. All the hassles of the past 24 hours were forgiven. This bionic diabetic was in rapture.

Over the next six weeks of testing, I came down to earth as I realized that while the sensor enabled me to drastically cut my usual number of lows, it did not eliminate them. One problem was that the sensor was simply not as accurate as a blood-glucose tester. Medtronic's studies showed the sensor's accuracy could be off by as much as 18 percent. None of the other sensors approved by the FDA were as accurate as a good old-fashioned blood-sugar test either. And often I found my Real-Time sensor to be almost laughably far off the number measured by my meter.

But even if the sensor's readings were perfect, a bigger problem loomed: I still had to decide how to use them in deciding how much insulin to take and how much food to eat. At times the flood of numbers pouring forth from the sensor could get overwhelming, requiring more attention and thought than I might be able or willing to give. Even when I did give it my full attention, deciding how much insulin to take based on a sugar level rising from 150 to 180 over a 20-minute period while a plateful of spaghetti was about to be served after munching on a few slices of French bread was akin to using pure intuition to guess how much of a fuel thrust to give a missile in hopes of hitting a postage stamp in Panama.

Plus, three of my sensor catheters slipped out during my six-week test and required early replacement, which would have been especially annoying had I been paying the $35 that each sensor costs; I wasn't, because Medtronic had supplied everything free for testing.

Despite all the hassles, there was one huge, undeniable benefit: during the entire time I used the sensor, I had only a few lows that left me feeling woozy, the kind I usually put up with two or three times every week (sometimes two or three times in a single day).

On the other hand, the greatest weakness of the continuous glucose sensor proved to be its greatest asset: its *continuousness*. The darn thing is always at you, beeping, vibrating, beckoning you to check it, like a BlackBerry. Sure, knowledge is power; it puts you in "control," with a constant information feed. There you are, at the helm of your diabetes! It's just you and your blood sugars, *mano-a-mano*.

But let's get real. Yeah, okay, the sensor is useful. But it's maddening. It offers not liberation from blood sugars, but a kind of enslavement to them. It might be high-tech, but it's not the diabetic's equivalent of a jet pack. It's more like a pair of wings, with instructions for flapping.

PSYCHOLOGICAL TOLL

Just to be clear, the incessant demands for self-monitoring and self-control that are placed upon people with diabetes, and that are only increased by high-tech gadgetry, have real consequences for their mental health. At the 2009 annual meeting of the American Diabetes Association, researchers from the University of Colorado Health Science Center reported a startling finding: compared to people who do not have diabetes, *depression is twice as common among people with type 1*. Among 458 adults with type 1 diabetes, a whopping 32.1 percent met the criteria for depression on the Beck Depression Inventory, compared to 16.0 percent of those without diabetes. What's more, just over 20 percent of people with type 1 were taking an antidepressant medication, compared to only 12.1 percent of those without diabetes.

In a particularly vicious circle, people with diabetes who do experience depression are at increased risk of forgoing their insulin injections and their self-testing, which in turn makes them feel worse. Women in particular have been known to react to all the dietary pressures with eating disorders, including one called "diabulimia," in which they intentionally reduce the amount of insulin they take in order to lose weight, even though doing so immediately causes all the symptoms of uncontrolled diabetes, including frequent urination, thirst, and exhaustion. A recent study by Joslin researchers found that a remarkable 30 percent of young women engaged in such behaviors, even though doing so *tripled their risk of death* over an 11-year period.

To find out more about the kind of emotional issues that can lead to such behavior, I met with 20-year-old Maggy Walsh near her hometown of Sudbury, Massachusetts (one of the Boston suburbs afflicted with a high rate of type 1). For our meeting place, she chose, of all places, Lizzy's Homemade Ice Cream Shop in downtown Waltham.

"Most of my friends who have diabetes have some sort of anxiety issues," said the pretty young blonde with a nose ring and a silver stud above her lip. Having attended and served as a counselor at the Clara Barton camp for diabetics for most of the eight summers since she'd developed diabetes, she was in as good a position as anyone to see how diabetes continues to affect young people despite, or because of, tight control.

"I honestly believe that there is something about the combination of being a teenage girl and having diabetes that just makes life infinitely more difficult," she told me. "Most of the girls I know who've had diabetes through puberty have really struggled with some form of depression, anxiety, even self-mutilation or diabulimia. My best friend had the diabulimic behaviors when she'd get depressed. And another good friend has been dealing with it for years. Her last A1C was 13 or 14. She's a wonderful, very intelligent, kind, loving person. And she knows that not taking her insulin is bad. But at some point it's like any other mental disorder, and it becomes an obsession, an addiction, to take that control. Her sugars got so high, she ended up in a coma for a month. She was on a respirator. Her parents and siblings thought she was going to die, but she survived."

And what about Maggy herself? "I've been really frustrated ever since my friend lapsed into that coma. It's made me angry and bitter. I feel it's so unfair. My friends are wonderful people. They're caring, they're intelligent. They're doing great things with their lives. It's not right that they have to deal with that."

At times, Maggy said, she's thrown her pump across the room, or taken a syringe and angrily jabbed at a vein on her leg or abdomen in order to cause a large bruise. And the worst of it, she said, is knowing that no matter how hard she tries to control her diabetes, "At least once a day, I'll feel bad, from either a low or a high. What really kills me is working with these four-year-olds at the Clara Barton camp, and knowing they're going to feel like shit once a day for the rest of their lives."

THE BIG FIX

Of course, nobody ever said that tight control or its accoutrements—pumps, test strips, and sensors—were a cure. The cure, we have been told since the early 1970s, would come from a transplant of the insulin-producing islet cells. Back in 1972, biologists from Washington University in St. Louis first reported success in curing diabetes by transplanting islets—but only in rats. In humans, the procedure turned out to be a bust; even with heavy doses of antirejection drugs, most islets simply died. For years, reports of new approaches, such as encapsulating the islets inside tiny bubbles, would come and go.

Then, in June of 2000, a major breakthrough was reported in the *New England Journal of Medicine*. Using a combination of three antirejection drugs—Zenapax, Rapamune, and Prograf—a team at the University of Edmonton in Alberta, Canada, found what appeared to be the magic formula: of seven patients who received transplanted islets, all had normal blood-sugar levels, without the need for insulin injections, after one year. The so-called Edmonton Protocol became an immediate sensation among researchers and the media. Even *The New Yorker* published an article lauding the treatment in 2003.

And then the other shoe dropped. "Diabetes Treatment Fails to Live Up to Promise," ran the headline in the *New York Times* in September of 2006. Although most transplant recipients remained free of insulin injections after one year, after two years 86 percent needed to go back on the needle, researchers had found. Soon evidence emerged that the antirejection drugs used in the treatment could cause severe kidney damage. Other complications seen included weight gain, uncontrollable mouth sores, increased susceptibility to infections, and a heightened risk of cancer. Researchers began calling for an end to the procedure except in extraordinary circumstances.

"I think it should be stopped," said Dr. David Nathan, the leader of the DCCT study, when I visited his office in Boston. Referring to colleagues at Massachusetts General Hospital, he said, "We've done, oh, fifteen islet transplants. At one point we were the fourth busiest in the country, but we pulled back. We know those islets die over several years. It has to be considered experimental. On balance, after a lot of effort and thousands of these procedures done internationally, it seems pretty clear it's not ready for prime time."

Still, other physicians and researchers insist that the transplants should continue, as have many patients who received islet transplants under the Edmonton Protocol.

"For about four years, I was able to function as a normal non-diabetic," said Bob Teskey, 62, when I reached him by telephone at his home in Edmonton. "I had normal insulin function. I could eat what I wanted." Even though he now has to take injections again, the amount of insulin he takes is only about half as much as he needed before the procedure, which he underwent in 1999. "There's no doubt this was experimental. There's no doubt there is much work to be done. But the reality is I got four years of freedom."

More recently, Gayle Driediger, 50, underwent an islet transplant in 2008, knowing full well that it would probably result in only a temporary respite from insulin injections. "Being able to stop taking insulin injections altogether, even if only for a few years, was just overwhelming," she told me. "My husband, daughter, and I all cried the first evening." She bridled at the view that the procedures should be stopped except under rare, experimental circumstances. "How to control my diabetes should be my own decision. There is no way I would say the operation wasn't worth it. It's beautiful. I love it."

Still, with only a few thousand human pancreases available each year in the United States for the procedure, at most it will be a rare, costly, and temporary fix, carrying significant medical risks—certainly not the "cure" that the research community has held it out to be for decades.

BACK TO WESTON

Around the same time that success with the first islet transplant in rats was reported, in the early 1970s, other researchers were making breakthroughs in establishing what causes type 1 diabetes. First came reports, in 1973 and 1974, that many people with type 1 had variations in certain genes that code for the immune system. Also in 1974, other studies showed that if white blood cells from people with type 1 diabetes were placed in a test tube with islet cells, the white blood cells attacked the islet cells. Since then, the prevailing orthodoxy, supported by hundreds of studies, has become that type 1 diabetes is an autoimmune disease, in which infection-fighting immune cells mistakenly target and attack their own body's islet cells as foreign. Indeed, researchers are now able to perform blood tests on seemingly healthy children that can predict with 50 percent to 90 percent accuracy their likelihood of developing type 1 in the next few years, based solely on the presence of "autoantibodies"—specialized white blood cells that have molecular markers indicating that they are, in fact, dead set on killing islets.

There is no question that an autoimmune attack does occur in most (but not quite all) people who develop type 1. The problem with this prevailing paradigm is that it tells us *how* diabetes occurs, through the destruction of islets by white blood cells, but not *why*. It says nothing about *what,* aside from a genetic predisposition, actually sets off the autoimmune attack. Nor does it tell us anything about places *where* type 1 diabetes has been increasing, reaching levels in many communities unimaginable a generation ago.

Which brings us back to Weston, Massachusetts.

Since the initial outbreak occurred during the 2007–08 school year, when seven children were diagnosed with type 1 diabetes within a two-mile radius, three more children were diagnosed in the same area in the early months of 2009. As Ann Marie Kreft, whose son Gus was one of the first diagnosed in the recent cluster, put it, "We now have ten diagnoses in a two-mile radius in twenty-four months."

To place those figures in context, a recent study in the journal *Diabetes* was entitled "The Rise of Childhood Type 1 Diabetes in the 20th Century." The paper noted that back in 1890, the reported annual death rate from diabetes for children under the age of 15 was 1.3 per 100,000 children in the United States. Because any death due to diabetes in those days surely had to be caused by what we now call type 1, researchers consider the 1.3 per 100,000 figure to be a rough estimate of the yearly incidence of new cases at that time. In Denmark, the rate was fairly similar, about 2 per 100,000 at the beginning of the 20th century. From that baseline, things took off. As the study states: "The best evidence available suggests that childhood diabetes showed a stable and relatively low incidence over the first half of the 20th century, followed by a clear increase that began at some time around or soon after the middle of the century." By the mid-1980s, the yearly incidence of new cases of type 1 had jumped to 14.8 per 100,000 children in Colorado. By the opening years of the 21st century, the incidence rate in six geographic areas of the United States, as measured in a new study run by the CDC, had climbed to 23.6 per 100,000 among non-Hispanic white children. "The incidence of type 1 diabetes in non-Hispanic white youth in the U.S. is one of the highest in the world," the study concluded. The rates were 68 percent higher than those reported in Colorado in the 1980s, and more than twice as high as reported in Philadelphia in the 1990s, the study noted.

Can it really be that rates of type 1 are now more than ten times higher than they were 100 years ago? According to Dr. Pina Imperatore, the chief epidemiologist in the diabetes division at the CDC, it's important to recognize that reported rates in the past are subject to uncertainties. But, she said, "It seems the trend we're seeing in the United States today is similar to what has been reported in Europe and worldwide, about a 3 percent increase annually in the incidence of type 1."

While a 3 percent gain per year might not sound like much, imagine what would happen if you held onto a stock that gained 3 percent every year for a century. Through the magic of compound interest, it would produce a one-third overall gain in a decade—no great shakes, perhaps—but would be up 80 percent after two decades, 438 percent over a half century, and nearly 20-fold in 100 years.

What does that mean for Weston, or for any other town or neighborhood concerned about an apparent outbreak? While the CDC's new study, called SEARCH, is tracking incidence rates in six communities around the country, no national study is tracking rates as they occur elsewhere. In response to the CDC's recent SEARCH findings, however, a 2007 editorial in the *Journal of the American Medical Association* called for "a coordinated approach for childhood diabetes surveillance (i.e., mandated case-reporting). Only then can society respond effectively to the serious and increasing challenge of diabetes in youth."

According to Suzanne Condon, the associate commissioner and director of Environmental Health at the Massachusetts Department of Public Health, her preliminary statistics indicate that the rate of type 1 diabetes is some 30 percent higher in Massachusetts than the rate the CDC has seen nationwide. "I have a philosophy that if you don't look you'll never find," Dr. Condon told me. "Diabetes is one of these diseases that, right now, we need to be looking at it."

Whatever the exact rate of increase in the incidence of type 1 may be, this much is clear: it's rising, and no amount of test strips, insulin pumps, sensors, or islet-cell transplants will do anything to stop the rise. Rather than plugging the leak in the boat, we have been bailing out with teaspoons, all the while sinking deeper. In Part 2 of this book, we shall examine the five leading hypotheses that seek to explain what the source of this leak is, and how we might plug it.

But first, let's pick back up the *other* thread of our story: the rise of type 2 diabetes.

CHAPTER 4

The Sweetest Place on Earth

Type 2 Reaches Unimagined Heights: 1984 to the Present Day

R ANDY AND SUSIE BLANKENSHIP live along Buffalo Creek Road in Logan County, West Virginia—the county with the highest rate of type 2 diabetes in the United States, according to the Centers for Disease Control and Prevention. Just miles from their home, Buffalo Creek was the site of a notorious disaster on February 26, 1972, when a dam holding back coal slurry broke, setting loose a 30-foot wall of blackened waste water that killed 125 people, injured over 1,000, and left more than 4,000 homeless. The floodwaters had flowed over the site on which Randy later built his family's home in the early 1980s.

Their home is beautifully built and beautifully furnished, "country" in the style of *Country Living*, and wouldn't look out of place on any suburban street. Inside the two-car garage is a gorgeous red vintage pickup with a swirling "bowling ball" paint job on the hood, and a spotless all-terrain vehicle the Blankenships use for driving around the hills and hollows.

I had met the Blankenships the night before, at a diabetes support group, where I learned that Randy and all ten of his siblings have type 2 diabetes. Now I joined them at their kitchen table, where they sat with their daughter, Mishalla, as well as Mishalla's husband and young son, sharing a double-crust stuffed pizza with sausage that they'd ordered for dinner.

"I never had a weight problem, even after we started having children, until we moved here, closer to Randy's family," said Susie, who is of average weight now, after having undergone bariatric surgery a few years earlier. "Some people eat to live; they live to eat. You name it, they like it. When we have our family reunion, they have fried chicken, baked chicken, macaroni salad, chicken and dumplings, hot dogs on the grill, green beans with bacon fat in them. And all kinds of desserts. His mother, I can remember she would just eat sweets all the time. She loved 'em. Loved sweets."

The little boy played with a package of cookies on the table, then reached for a box of Junior Mints.

"Eat your candy," said his father. "Eat 'em."

"He loves those little things," said Mishalla.

Randy told me how he succeeded in losing 50 pounds: by joining in a family bet to see who could lose the most. "If you lost weight you didn't have to pay the money," he said. "I beat them all."

Dinner over, Randy and Susie walked next door to the double-width trailer in which his youngest sister, Tammy, lives with her 18-year-old son, Jeremy. Another sister, Vicky, was visiting from Lexington, Kentucky. Jeremy's 17-year-old girlfriend, Ashley, had also dropped by.

We sat down in the living room, which had a large-screen TV, a glass case displaying Tammy's collection of Christmas dolls, and a portable, plastic toilet seat with metal support rails. Tammy perched on the edge of the hospital bed in which she sleeps, dangling her feet, mottled purple and missing two toes (amputated due to circulatory problems caused by diabetes). Still retaining a girlishness about her, with short brown hair and only slightly overweight, she commenced to tell her story.

"I've known about my diabetes for twenty-two years, since I was twenty-six," she began.

"I had just turned thirty-one when I got it," piped in her blond, blue-eyed sister, Vicky, also dressed in a nightgown.

"I've had it about five years," said Randy. "I was probably about forty-eight."

"I think that's because he's a man, and he exercises more," commented Vicky.

"I stay busy from daylight to dark," agreed Randy.

"It's hard for me to keep up with him," said Jeremy.

Things had gone reasonably well for Tammy, she explained, until about ten years earlier, when she began drastically cutting back on her insulin and other medications in order to lose weight. "I had a husband seven years younger than me," she said. "I was married to him for twenty-three years. I tried to keep him happy. So I was destroying myself for him."

"That's why she's in the shape's she's in, my opinion," said her son. "It was like six years she wouldn't take her pills."

Her husband eventually left her anyway, for the home aide who had been caring for her. Ironically enough, Tammy said, "His new wife is two times my size. That was my birthday gift three years ago, when the divorce was finalized on my birthday."

She returned to taking her medications as prescribed, but continued eating whatever she liked. "I used to be bad about it. If I wanted to eat a bag of candy, I'd eat a bag of candy. I was on fifteen different pills until I started kidney dialysis. It's been about a month and a half now. They've taken me off some of my medications."

I asked Randy how many drugs he takes. "Oh son," he sighed, and launched into a list that would have been ridiculous if it weren't so appalling. "I take aspirin. Glucophage. Lipitor. Quinaretic. Crestor. Tricor. Glipizide. Actos. Exforge. Dynacirc."

"I have five children," said Vicky, "and all of them have high cholesterol, high blood pressure, high triglycerides, and have to have their sugars checked quite often. They're already picking up all the symptoms."

I asked Tammy whether, instead of cutting back on her insulin to lose weight, she had ever considered bariatric surgery.

"My insurance won't pay for it," she said. "I've had several of my doctors even write me prescriptions that I needed the gastric bypass. But my insurance won't do it. I had a heart attack. Four or five months back I had a stent put in."

"I would rather have had the stomach surgery five years back, and die on the table," said Vicky, "instead of taking medicine until I'm seventy but suffered all this time."

"Every day we suffer," said Tammy. "Every day we suffer." Lowering her head into her hands, she continued, "It's destroyed my life. I don't go nowhere except to dialysis. This is my life right now," she said, patting the hospital bed.

"The pills. The suffering," said Vicky. And as if responding to how people might judge her sister, she added, "Nobody knows what other people feel like. They shouldn't try to judge somebody else's life. I go to three different doctors. I cleaned houses for seventeen years after I got my kids all raised. I worked up until just a few months ago. Now I take eighteen different prescriptions. Sometimes I just lay on my couch in pain."

Finally there was nothing more to say. I thanked them for sharing their stories and rose to leave. "Are those Barbie dolls?" I asked Tammy of the collection she had behind the glass display case. They reminded me of my daughter's "Holiday Barbie" dolls.

"Those are angels," she said. "They're like Christmas tree toppers. I used to have more of 'em. I love my angels."

DRUG MARKET RISING

How has it come to this? Perhaps, if we look back to the period in the mid-1980s, when only a handful of drugs were available for the treatment of type 2, and trace it forward to today, we can find the moment when we crossed over to the point of having too many drugs and not enough healing.

The battle over Orinase—the drug that had been launched to such great fanfare back in the late 1950s as the first pill for diabetes, then ran into trouble with the UGDP study in 1970, showing that it actually increased the risk of death—didn't end until 1984. During that period, some have estimated, Orinase and other sulfonylureas caused tens of thousands of deaths among the people taking them. The drugs' supporters, of course, continued to strongly dispute such estimates. But with Upjohn's exclusive patent rights finally expiring for Orinase, the company lost the motivation to continue the fight. And so, beginning in 1984, Orinase and other sulfonylureas were required by the FDA to carry, in boldface, a "SPECIAL WARNING ON INCREASED RISK OF CARDIOVASCULAR MORTALITY" on the labeling information that comes with every prescription. The warning states (it remains to this day on the labels of all sulfonylureas) that although controversies remain about the interpretation of the UGDP, the study's findings nevertheless "provide an adequate basis" for warning consumers about the possible cardiovascular risks associated with sulfonylureas. Yet most doctors continued to prescribe them, especially a second generation of sulfonylureas that were far more powerful than Orinase and Diabinese but carried the same warning.

Not surprisingly, when a bumper crop of new sugar-lowering drugs started to hit the market in the 1990s—the golden age of development for type 2 drugs—doctors and patients grabbed them with two fists. First came the approval in 1994 of metformin, a chemical cousin of phenformin (which was banned back in 1977 due to rare but potentially fatal side effects). Metformin was considered especially valuable because it did not cause dangerously low blood-sugar levels and tended to result in weight *loss* rather than weight *gain*. Sold under the brand name Glucophage, it eventually became the best-selling drug for type 2 diabetes and is a mainstay of treatment to this day, still considered by many physicians to be the safest and most effective pill to prescribe newly diagnosed patients.

The next big drug to hit the market, Rezulin, was vaunted as a potential blockbuster by its maker, Warner-Lambert, and given fast-track approval by the FDA in January of 1997. It caused a little weight gain and worked directly against insulin resistance in the muscles, meaning that the body actually needs less insulin to maintain normal sugar levels. By that fall, however, dozens of patients taking Rezulin were hospitalized with liver ailments, some of whom died. The liver toxicity proved enough to convince regulators in Britain to ban the drug on December 1 of that year, but in the United States, the FDA decided that a warning to doctors to check patients' liver function was a sufficient response. In March of 1999, however, the FDA acknowledged that 43 cases of liver failure, including 28 deaths, had been linked to Rezulin. That same month, David J. Graham, MD, a senior epidemiologist at the agency, called Rezulin among the most dangerous drugs on the market. Still the leadership of the FDA defended it.

In January of 2000, Robert I. Misbin, MD, a senior medical officer at the FDA who had previously supported approval of the drug, began calling for its withdrawal from the U.S. market in private emails to his colleagues. When his correspondence was published two months later in the *Los Angeles Times* (in a series of articles that eventually won the Pulitzer prize for investigative reporting), Misbin was threatened with dismissal.

The same series of articles soon revealed that another FDA medical officer, John L. Gueriguian, MD, had originally been in charge of reviewing the drug back in 1996, and had recommended that it be rejected due to concerns that it could harm the liver and the heart. Gueriguian, it turned out, had been removed from the assignment following pressure from Warner-Lambert; his recommendation against approval had been struck from the official FDA record and withheld from an advisory committee. Furthermore, a St. Louis physician who had supervised some of the early clinical trials for Warner-Lambert was now charging that the company had "deliberately omitted reports of liver toxicity and misrepresented serious adverse events experienced by patients in their clinical studies."

When the FDA finally announced on March 21, 2000, that it was banning Rezulin, the numbers racked up during its three years on the market were impressive, on two very different levels. On the one hand, it had earned Warner-Lambert $2.1 billion; on the other, it was suspected in 391 deaths. Even so, by then, two other drugs, Actos and Avandia, had already been approved under the same fast-track process that had led to Rezulin's approval.

MORE DRUGS, MORE RISKS

By 2007, people with type 2 diabetes had a mind-boggling array of 18 different sugar-lowering drugs and three combination products to choose from. What they did not have was clear and convincing proof that any of them protect against the development of heart disease, the leading complication of diabetes, or that using them aggressively to achieve tight control of their sugar levels would extend their lives.

That began to change on June 14, 2007, when Steven Nissen, MD, a prominent cardiologist at the Cleveland Clinic, published an analysis in the *New England Journal of Medicine* of Avandia, one of the drugs given fast-track approval back in 1999. By combining data from previously published studies, as well as from databases maintained by the FDA and the drug's manufacturer, GlaxoSmithKline, he found that, compared to patients not taking the drug, type 2 patients taking Avandia had a 43 percent increased risk of heart attack and a 64 percent increased risk of death due to cardiovascular causes.

The findings provoked skepticism from diabetes specialists who pointed out that a meta-analysis cannot provide convincing proof of anything, because it mashes up previous studies into a hash. Nissen, in fact, agreed with his critics, arguing only that the study pointed out the need for carefully constructed, randomized trials to resolve the matter one way or the other. The FDA, he said, needed to begin requiring that all diabetes drugs be studied for their effects on the heart.

If the Nissen meta-analysis was a hand grenade, the next study to hit, on February 7, 2008, was a bombshell. The Action to Control Cardiovascular Risk in Diabetes (ACCORD) study had been expressly designed by the National Heart, Lung and Blood Institute to test the tight-control hypothesis in people with type 2 diabetes, to see whether near-normal sugars would not merely prevent complications of the eyes, kidneys, and nerves, but would actually prevent heart attacks and stroke in those considered at high risk for such complications. The study was huge, involving over 10,000 people with type 2, and it was supposed to run for over five years. Patients in the tight-control group aimed to keep their A1C levels below 6, meaning that their sugar levels would be in the non-diabetic range. To achieve that, some had to test their sugar levels as often as eight times a day and take up to three sugar-lowering medications.

But 18 months before it was to have been completed, researchers stopped the study early after finding exactly the *opposite* of what they had expected: 257 patients in the tight-control group had died, compared to 203 in the standard-treatment group, a statistically significant difference. The president of the American College of Cardiology called the findings "confusing and disturbing." After all, the guidelines of both the ADA and the American Association of Clinical Endocrinologists called for keeping sugars as low as possible—a strategy that now appeared to increase the risk of heart attack and death.

Some comfort came later that year, when another large study, known as ADVANCE, found no increased risk of death or heart attack in tight-control patients with average A1Cs of 6.5, compared to the standard-control group with an average A1C of 7.3. Then again,

ADVANCE found no benefit either for tight control on the risk of death or heart attacks.

And another large study, the Veterans Affairs Diabetes Trial, likewise found no benefit of tight control in reducing the risk of heart attack, stroke, or other cardiovascular events; the only demonstrable effect of tight control, VADT found, was an increase in the risk of experiencing hypoglycemia.

On the other hand, the United Kingdom Prospective Diabetes Study found that 10 years after patients had completed the type 2 study, those who had been on the tight control regimen had a 15 percent lower risk of suffering a heart attack, and a 13 percent lower risk of dying from any cause, than those on standard control. Those who had taken metformin had enjoyed even greater benefits of tight control: a 33 percent lower risk of heart attack and 27 percent lower risk of death due to any cause.

Still, the negative results of the ACCORD, ADVANCE, and VA studies could not be ignored. By the summer of 2008, it was clear that something was amiss with the FDA's approach of approving so many drugs for type 2 based solely on their ability to lower blood sugars, without demanding proof of their effects on heart disease and overall life expectancy. In early July, the FDA scheduled a meeting of its diabetes drug advisory committee to consider the matter.

It took until after lunch on the first day for Steven Nissen, the doctor who had started the whole brouhaha with his meta-analysis of Avandia, to make the case that cardiovascular testing of diabetes drugs was not only sensible and practical but long overdue.

"Here we are, 50 years after the initial introduction of anti-diabetic agents," Nissen said. "And although cardiovascular disease is the cause of death in 75 percent of diabetics, there exists no well-designed, adequately powered, comparative effectiveness trials evaluating macrovascular outcomes [heart attacks and strokes] for diabetes drugs. We have a knowledge gap. There are certainly many ways to lower blood sugar. What we really need to know are what agents improve health outcomes, and what agents can we develop beyond current therapies that will improve health outcomes."

Nissen then tweaked the endocrinologists in the room by coining a name for a "disorder" that he called "glucose-centricity." "It's the irrational belief," Nissen said, "that lowering blood sugar using virtually any pharmacological means will produce a reliable reduction in adverse outcomes. I think what we've learned in the last year is that that's not correct. And so we've got to move beyond a glucose-centric approach. We have drugs to lower blood sugar. You know, people are not dying out there because we can't figure out how to lower their blood sugar. We have 10 classes of drugs to lower blood sugar. We need ways to lower blood sugar that reduce the complications."

Eight days before Christmas, on December 17, 2008, the FDA announced a new policy, effective immediately, requiring that before any new drug for type 2 diabetes is approved, evidence must be presented that it will not increase the risk of heart attacks, strokes, or other cardiovascular events.

NO EXIT?

If sugar-lowering pills for type 2 diabetes carry so many risks, why do so many people with type 2 take them? Why don't they just eat less, exercise more, and make their diabetes disappear? Why don't they read one of those books about "miracle" diets that supposedly cure diabetes in four weeks, and be done with it?

Excellent question. And if you're a person with type 2, or a doctor who works with them, you know the answer: because sticking to a diet-and-exercise plan closely enough to lose—*and keep off!*—enough pounds to reverse diabetes is just very, very, *very* hard for the average person. It's not that diets and exercise don't work. They do, if you stick to them. At least they do in the early stages of the disease, but as type 2 progresses, even the toughest diet rarely reverses it. As Professor Paul Zimmet of the International Diabetes Institute in Melbourne,

Australia, stated at a diabetes meeting in Rome in 2008: "Lifestyle may work, but the only place it may work is Alcatraz."

Actually, Zimmet was being a bit of a cynic there. In 2001, the largest study ever conducted to test the ability of diet and exercise to *prevent* diabetes (which is a different matter, by the way, than reversing it) proved to be a smashing success. Once again, the doctor who led the study was David Nathan, who led the DCCT involving tight control for people with type 1 diabetes. He and colleagues at 27 medical centers around the country enrolled 3,234 people and assigned them to receive metformin, a placebo, or a lifestyle program involving classes and coaches who kept track of their progress. The lifestyle program, the study found after three years, cut the participants' risk of developing diabetes by more than half—an even better result, by the way, than metformin had. As Nathan told the *New York Times:* "We weren't asking them to train for a marathon. They're a bunch of pretty normal people who are at a high risk for diabetes. We didn't grow them in a test tube. What we asked them to do, in the end, was not overwhelming. I don't see this as out of reach for the 10 million people who are at high risk for diabetes."

Fantastic. So how have we done with that?

Back in 1975, you might recall, an estimated 10 million people had type 2 diabetes, half of whom had been diagnosed by a doctor, another half as yet undiagnosed. By 1993, the total number had climbed to about 14 million. By 2001, the year Dr. Nathan's lifestyle study was released, the figure had reached 16 million. Since then, the figure has climbed by nearly 50 percent, to 23.6 million in 2009, according to the CDC. That's 7.8 percent of the entire population. For people ages 60 and over, *nearly one in four* currently have diabetes.

From a purely practical viewpoint, it should be clear by now to anyone willing to face up to reality that diets and exercise programs will simply not work in enough people, enough of the time, to stop the rate of type 2 from continuing its upward trajectory, or even to reverse it. Not that each individual shouldn't try his or her best in the meanwhile.

I myself jog regularly (although not as often as I always intend) and work hard to manage my diet, insulin and blood-sugar levels. The point is, though, that for the larger medical community to continue to expect that individual diet and exercise programs will turn around the type 2 pandemic amounts to willful indifference to the facts.

Of course, it would be ridiculous and offensive to suggest—and I am not suggesting—that all the advancements in care for diabetes over the past century have been for naught, or that dietitians don't help a lot of people. Even the staunchest consumer-protection groups would concede that only a handful of the many drugs sold for type 2 diabetes have been associated with controversial findings of risky side effects. Most do the job as advertised: they lower sugar levels, safely and effectively. One of my own brothers, diagnosed with type 2 a couple of years ago, now takes metformin and is doing well with it. And I'm always glad to hear when he tells me that he's walking to work or trying a new diet. Moreover, the drugs and the diets do lower the risk of many complications. Rates of retinopathy, kidney failure, nerve damage, and lower-extremity amputations have all declined markedly among diabetics since the mid-1990s.

Still, according to the CDC, diabetes remains the leading cause of new cases of blindness among adults, kidney failure, kidney dialysis, and non-traumatic lower-extremity amputations. And overall, the risk of death among people with diabetes is about twice that of people without the disease.

Is this what progress looks like?

Before moving on to investigate whether there might be other, more effective ways to get hold of the diabetes pandemic—to actually *prevent* people from getting diabetes, rather than just lecturing them to lose weight, or giving them pills if the diets fail—let's end this first section of the book, which has traced the disease's epic rise from obscurity, by taking a closer look at Logan County, where the Blankenhships live.

WORST-CASE SCENARIO

In June of 2008, for the first time ever, the CDC released county-by-county breakdowns of diabetes rates across the United States. It was then that I figured out that the highest rate of diabetes in the entire country, according to the numbers on the CDC's website, was Logan County, where 14.8 percent of everyone over the age of 20 has been diagnosed with it. That's well over double the rate of diagnosed diabetes in the rest of the country.

Uncertain whether I was reading the CDC's figures correctly, since they didn't actually include a "top ten" list, I called the agency to double-check that Logan County really is number one.

"I come to the same conclusion," said Edward Gregg, PhD, chief of the epidemiology and statistics branch of the CDC's Division of Diabetes, when I reached him by telephone. He emphasized, however, that the estimate falls within a statistical ballpark, or "confidence interval," with 95 percent confidence that the true rate is no lower than 11.7 percent and no higher than 18.6 percent. "The truth is probably somewhere between the confidence interval we give," he said. "The reality may be that some county in Mississippi is actually a bit higher than Logan County. But these are our best estimates to date. Methodologically this is a huge step beyond what we've ever had before."

Satisfied that Logan's rate is as high as anywhere in America, I made plans to visit there the last week of October 2008, to see why all the pills and injections and lifestyle advice weren't working, and just to be there in diabetic hell on Halloween.

Among the many statistics I gleaned about the county, one jumped out: the average lifespan of women in Logan County actually *dropped* by two years between 1989 and 1999, and is now the 16th-shortest life expectancy for women in the nation. Even so, local health officials reached by telephone before my departure did not seem very concerned.

"I honestly think we have a very good program," said Peggy Addams, a nurse and certified diabetes educator who runs the West Virginia Diabetes Prevention and Control Program in Charleston. For her, diabetes is personal: she and her husband both have it, as do two of her brothers. One of the factors working against the people in Logan County, she said, is the lack of sidewalks for walking. "Your suburb probably has sidewalks," she told me. "We don't have those. When you get to Logan County, you'll find that sidewalks are very few and far between. We have coal trucks running on relatively narrow roads. It doesn't really allow for safe walking."

I made three calls to the Logan County Health Department to reach its only physician, who is scheduled to work there on Friday mornings, but who was away each time I called. I finally reached the health officer, Livia N. Cabauatan, MD, at her private practice. "We're doing pretty well in Logan," she said. "We did a diabetic screening clinic less than a month ago. We had a very good turnout. Almost one hundred people came. Some of them don't have doctors. We gave them all free glucose monitors, with the help of the drug companies that came over and gave them to us."

On the website of the one hospital in the county, Logan Regional Medical Center, no endocrinologists or other diabetes specialists were listed among the 74 physicians on staff. In fact, I learned, there is not a single endocrinologist in the entire county. I called Logan Regional and was put through to the office of the chief administrator, Kevin Fowler. His assistant, Sammy Cook, said that Mr. Fowler didn't have time to discuss the matter. "You'd probably want to talk to an internist who treats diabetes," Sammy said. "We have several. Most of them are foreign. They're hard to understand. Dr. Radha is best informed." I called the office of Dr. Radha Kukkillaya, but the receptionist there said he wasn't available, and suggested I just swing by to speak with him for a few minutes when I arrived in town.

SUPPORT GROUP

Early in the evening on Tuesday, October 28, I found myself nego-
tiating treacherous Route 10, a switchback roller coaster of a road,
with a 50-foot drop down to the Guyandotte River on my right and
coal-seamed cliffs looming on the left. Strip-mining scooper trucks
could be glimpsed high atop the mountain, their lights piercing eerily
through smoke and dust. Arriving in the small town of Man just past
6 P.M., I made my way to the Community Health Foundation, a modest
medical clinic, where the only diabetic support group in the county
was scheduled to have its monthly meeting.

"I don't know why so few came tonight," said the nurse who leads
the group, Joanne Klein, when I joined her and the evening's attendees: an elderly couple and a grandmother accompanied by her young
grandson. "Usually we get more. I suppose it's kind of cold out."

At 59, Joanne was neatly dressed in a white jacket, green pants,
and white shoes. She flipped through laminated cards on a spiral
binder as she spoke to the group about foot care, important for diabetics because of the risk of amputation due to impaired circulation
and nerve function.

"Nails should be cut straight across," Joanne told them.

"Does it hurt to wear socks twenty-four hours a day?" asked 75-
year-old Winsel Elliott, seated beside his wife, Grace, age 70.

"No, that's fine," said Joanne. "So long as they're not too tight, cutting off circulation, that's fine."

"What scares me is my dad was a bad diabetic," Grace said after
Joanne had finished her presentation. "One of my sisters went completely blind from the sugar."

"My brother died at fifty-seven, he never followed his diet," said
Sue White, who wore a Winnie the Pooh sweatshirt over her ample
frame. "He ended up on kidney dialysis for three months. He went
blind. He had open heart surgery twice."

As Sue's young grandson literally spun himself dizzy on the deep-blue linoleum floor, a janitor came by with a buffer and we all stood to munch on the deli meats, cheeses, and bread that Joanne had brought.

"My daddy, once a week he had him a full gross of potatoes, he put in the lard—and he lived till eighty-eight years old," Winsel said as he prepared a sandwich. "You never heard about diabetes. They got up before daylight, fed their animals, then breakfast was ready, go to the fields. And I mean, around here, places I could show you, where they used to farm it, now the people don't even raise a garden."

"And the kids don't go out and play like they used to," said Joanne. "They sit inside and exercise their thumbs on the video games."

Hearing our conversation, the woman buffing the floor mentioned that she has diabetes, her husband has diabetes, and all ten of his brothers and sisters have diabetes too. Amazed, I asked if I could meet with her husband in the next few days.

"He's right in the other room, waiting to drive me home," she said.

With the support group breaking up, I said good night to Joanne and the others and followed the woman, who introduced herself as Susie Blankenship. Her husband, Randy, stood to shake hands and said he'd be happy to tell me about his family. Fifty-three years old, he weighed 272 pounds after losing 50 pounds on a diet. A former coal miner, on disability from a long-ago injury, Randy was bald, with a trim white beard and mustache, and the letters *RB, SB* tattooed on his arm. He and Sue, high school sweethearts, had been married since 1973, when Sue was just 16.

"My mom had diabetes, died of congestive heart failure," Randy said. "She was sixty-eight. Dad was seventy-two. All eleven of us kids got diabetes now. And all of us had open heart surgery but three. My brother Luther had two open heart surgeries. I'm the youngest brother of the family, but I'm the biggest. I take Byetta twice a day, but the other morning my sugar was sky high, it was 472."

I pointed out that a blood sugar that high, compared to a normal reading of 80, was nearly enough to send a person to a hospital.

"He just decided he was tired of watching what he ate," said Sue. "He stopped taking his medication."

"For six months I took nothing. It's a lifestyle you get tired of."

"One of his sisters lost two toes," said Sue. "She's bed-fast. She had to have hip surgery and never healed good. She's on kidney dialysis now. She's forty-eight, and she's been battling diabetes since her thirties."

That's when we made plans for me to visit them, as described in the opening of this chapter.

FAST FOOD RISING

On Wednesday morning, I drove over to Logan Regional Medical Center and found the ground-floor office of Dr. Radha, the internist whose receptionist had told me to stop by.

After spending half an hour waiting, I was told without explanation that neither he nor his partner would see me. I reminded the receptionist that the office of the hospital's chief administrator had referred me to him, and that I'd come all the way from New Jersey, but to no avail.

Uncertain how to proceed, I took to wandering the grounds of the medical office park surrounding the hospital, in search of any doctor who might be willing to speak. After being turned down twice more, I walked into the waiting room of Satyanarayana Mamidi, MD, a cardiologist, and after a brief wait was ushered into his office.

"We really don't need endocrinologists here," Dr. Mamidi told me after I asked him about the lack of specialists in America's most diabetic county. "General practitioners can take very good care of them. This community probably couldn't sustain an endocrinologist." He estimated that about half of his heart patients have diabetes, but said,

"Most are well taken care of by their primary-care physician." One of the best in the area, he said, was Dr. Kenneth Sells, an internist who happened to have diabetes himself.

Dr. Mamidi blamed the rise of diabetes in the area on the many fast-food restaurants that had sprung up since he and his wife had arrived from India 26 years earlier. (I later counted within the county's borders five Pizza Huts, five Wendy's, five Subways, three Taco Huts, three Gino's Pizzas, two KFCs, two Papa John's, two McDonald's, two Burger Kings, two Little Ceasars, one Blimpie, one Shoney's, one Arby's, and one Captain D's Seafood—a staggering 36 fast-food restaurants in a county of 37,710 people.)

"Believe it or not, when I came to Logan, there was no McDonald's," he said. "Wendy's just came in after I arrived. These fast-food restaurants have really grown in the last fifteen years."

A couple of hours later, at the local Bob Evans, I met Sandra Ooten, a nurse-practitioner and dietitian who has worked as a certified diabetes educator for 20 years.

"Can I get you biscuits with that?" asked the waitress after I had ordered a grilled-cheese sandwich and for Sandra a salad.

"I can understand why there's an epidemic of diabetes here," said Ooten, a middle-aged, bespectacled woman who, while not exactly thin, was thinner than any other adult I'd met in Logan so far. "There's very few women who cook around here anymore. The meal's out of a microwave or a drive-through. Call in and get a pizza, or go to fast food. It's not unusual for people to tell me they eat cold pizza for breakfast."

Born and raised in Logan County, Ooten thought she would save the world from diabetes and obesity when she started out. Then she ran into a wall of apathy, even hostility.

"I had an ADA-certified diabetes program in downtown Williamson, in the next county over," she told me. "It ended up closing. Couldn't get referrals. Doctors would not refer. They thought I'd steal their patients. Now I'm working with a physician who has a contract with Massey Energy, the big coal company here. All I see are coal miners. One young man, he's twenty years old, his weight was 376. I told him, 'I'm really concerned about your weight.' He said, 'Well, I just eat too much. I've been eating this, this, and this.' I proceeded to talk about the quantities, the food choices, the increased daily activity. I thought we were having a good conversation. The next day, my boss got a letter from his mother about me harassing him about his weight. And that's not unusual. I had an appointment with a nineteen-year-old boy. He was over 255. I told him I was concerned about his weight. He went outside to his mom. She said, 'What did she say?' He said, 'She told me I was fat.' And they laughed.

"If diabetes just hurt," Ooten said, "that person would be in my office within hours. If it just caused them the discomfort of a cold, they'd come. But sometimes I have to chase them down. I don't think anything will work until it is tied somehow to money, or their insurance. That seems to be the only thing to motivate people."

What did she make of the usual recommendations one hears at medical meetings for, say, teaching diabetics to count carbs?

"You can't take people who don't have a clue what a carb is, and then say, 'Now I want you to count every carb that goes in your mouth.' With these folks who tell me their typical dinner is two cheeseburgers and a big fries, sometimes I say, 'Can you get just one cheeseburger? Can you get a regular fry?' Even that seems to be something they can't do. The only thing worse than the epidemic is the apathy."

DEVIL'S NIGHT

The next day was October 30, when trick-or-treating was scheduled (yes, scheduled in advance, and listed in the newspaper) from 6 P.M. until 8 P.M. in the town of Man. Beforehand, I met with Anita Sedlock, supervisor of child nutrition for Logan County schools.

"Number one in the country?" she asked when I told her about the county's diabetes rate. "That's not a good number one to have." But, she said, the state and county were working hard to turn the problem around. "As of July first, the West Virginia Department of Education allowed nothing but one hundred percent juice, water, or milk sold in machines on school property. Not even diet soda. And no candy in the school. Right this week, parents want to bring cupcakes and they want to bring this and that. I threatened to take tomorrow off because of all the fussing from the parents about the rules. It's not the children who are the problem with the soda and candy machines, it's the parents."

The new policies, she said, go well beyond vending machines. "All fryers have been taken out of our schools, as of about a year ago. There's nothing deep fried. No corn dogs. French fries are baked." And all foods have to meet nutritional standards aimed at cutting obesity.

Glad to have met someone making a difference in the area, and with another two hours before trick-or-treating was scheduled to begin, I headed over to the office of another person with his thumb in the dyke: Dr. Kenneth Sells, the lone practitioner at Main Street Family Practice in Logan's desolate downtown. In his early fifties, slightly overweight, and plainly overworked, he stole ten minutes to speak with me while a dozen patients waited.

"What the problem is here," he began, "is that sixty percent of my patients are diabetics, and sixty percent of my practice is Medicare or Medicaid. Endocrinologists can't live on what Medicare pays, and the insurers will not pay me for diabetic education. They say that is the doctors' responsibility, to educate patients as they go along.

"What happens is, we're throwing medicines at them, but medication is not a cure. We're not getting at the core of diabetes, which is diet and exercise. Some people are taking six, eight pills for their diabetes, checking their sugars four times a day. They just hate it."

And then the harried physician lapsed into a kind of spontaneous poetry. "Diabetes is a child that you can't make stop crying. In the beginning you can rock it, you can pat it, you can change its diaper, you can feed it. But after a while, when you haven't had any sleep and it's still crying, you're ready to call it quits. The treatments are effective, for what they're worth. We can get someone's A1C to come down in three months. But they have to work so hard to do it. Think of diabetes as a chronic disease that you never get rid of, that you have to constantly fight. It's a fight you sometimes feel like fighting, and sometimes you don't."

How well did he treat his own diabetes? "Sometimes I'm too worried about my patients to worry about me," he confessed. "My head might be hurting because I haven't taken my shot yet, but there's someone who's been waiting three hours to see me in the waiting room. I can have a blood sugar of five hundred all day and not have time to bother with it. To me it's a nuisance."

Did he see any solution beyond lecturing his patients to eat less and prescribing them more pills? "We need programs here to say, if a car has pollution limits, and has to get so many miles per gallon, then food has to have some limits too. You cannot have a fast-food restaurant on every block, or have more than two portions in a single serving. Let's put some of the responsibility on the manufacturer rather than all of it on the consumer."

At 6 P.M., back on the main drag of South Man, I heard church bells peal as hundreds of trick-or-treaters crowded along the street. Homeowners sat on their front stoops, holding bags of candy for ghouls, witches, ninjas, and Spider-Men who walked with their parents, some of them looking to weigh 400 pounds or more. Walking past a Grim Reaper carrying a scythe, I found myself thinking that tonight, Devil's Night, the treats *were* the tricks.

ANOTHER NUMBER ONE

The next morning, at Logan Middle School, I saw that one of the main hallways was lined with posters made by the kids, comparing how their lives differed from their grandparents' lives.

"I like to surf the Internet, hang out with friends, go to movies," wrote one student. She quoted her grandmother as saying, "I watched black and white television or listened to the radio. But most of the time I played outside until dark and then we had to come inside."

On another poster, the child wrote, "I ride the bus or my mom takes me to school." His grandfather, on the other hand, said, "All the kids had to walk to school. There was no bus to ride. Even in the snow and rain we had to walk." The same child then wrote, "I have a few chores around the house. I have to keep my room clean, help with the laundry and sweep. Did you have any chores?" The grandfather's chores included carrying coal in for heat, mowing the lawn, and "I had to carry in water from the well for us to drink and for my mom to cook in and us to bathe in. We had to heat the water to bathe in so we had to bring in extra coal for that."

Another student wrote, "Nana was in the sixth grade in 1948. Eating: cooked at home and usually ate as a family. Now. We eat out a lot, at different times."

And another: "We have TV and video games for entertainment. What did you do for entertainment? Answer: We went outside to play games like kick the can or hide and go seek."

Driving out of town, I made one last stop, at the local Wal-Mart, to check out its grocery department. It turned out to be quite extensive, with plenty of fresh fruits and vegetables. Certainly anyone wanting inexpensive, healthy foods could find them here. But walking farther into the grocery section, I noticed a banner hanging over a display of Little Debbie snacks. Stacked up on the display case were boxes of Nutty Bars, Devil Creams, Iced Honey Buns, Donut Sticks, Coffee Cakes, Glazed Donuts, Frosted Donuts, Powdered Donuts, Boston Creme Rolls, Golden Cremes, Devil Squares, Strawberry Shortcake Rolls, Fancy Cakes, Chocolate Fudge Cakes, Zebra Cakes, Oatmeal Creme Pies, and Raisin Creme Pies. Across from the display was a Little Debbie poster showing a race-car driver. "Don't just stand there," it said, "Start snacking." And above the display case, a blue banner proclaimed: "Sweetest Store on Earth! Number One Wal-Mart in the World in Sales of Little Debbie Snack Cakes."

Heading home, north toward New Jersey, I had to wonder how long doctors would persist in looking for the causes of diabetes—and the reasons for its relentless rise—solely within the islets of Langerhans, rather than in the aisles of Wal-Mart.

THE REASONS

CHAPTER 5

The Accelerator Hypothesis

*Weight Gain as the Missing Link Between
Type 1 and Type 2*

TERRY WILKIN HAD HIS foot on the accelerator of his bright
orange 1976 Volkswagen camper van, his wife beside him and
their three kids in the backseat, as they drove through the Austrian Alps on a rainy day in August of 1986 when he was struck by a
Big Idea. It came to him so suddenly, in the classic "Eureka!" cliché
of science, that he nearly smashed down his foot on the brake in the
middle of the road. He didn't, so everyone was okay, but it would soon
become apparent that the orthodox view on what causes the two
kinds of diabetes, and why they are both increasing, had sustained
a major dent.

Wilkin's idea was as simple as it was heretical. As professor
of endocrinology and metabolism at Peninsula Medical School in
Plymouth, UK, and the editor of the respected scientific journal
Autoimmunology, he knew it offered a new answer to a fundamental
question that the field had supposedly answered more than half a
century earlier: Why do the fierce little warriors who constitute the
body's immune system not normally attack and destroy the body
itself, and what goes wrong when, in an autoimmune disease like

diabetes, they do? Here was a question of biology that even a poet or philosopher could love: How does the body distinguish between "self" and "non-self," between I and Thou? It might seem funny to think that the body doesn't automatically recognize itself. To us, looking at our hand on a table, or seeing our image in a mirror, self-recognition would seem . . . self-evident. Yet the self is not evident to the immune system without some molecular tricks.

The standard explanation, developed in the 1930s, is that every cell in the body is tagged with a "self" identifier—the molecular equivalent of a "do not disturb" sign on a hotel doorknob—and that when an attack nevertheless occurs, it's essentially because of a signaling problem, either with a misspelled sign placed on the cell's doorknob or a misreading of it by the immune system's roaming sentinels and warriors, known in polite circles as, ahem, white blood cells. By this view, nothing is actually wrong with the organ getting attacked; it's all the immune system's fault. To cure the autoimmune disease, it naturally follows, all one would have to do is to fix the faulty signals that have led to the errant attack on the body's own organs.

And that's just what diabetes researchers have been trying to do since the 1970s, when type 1 was proved to be an autoimmune disorder. So far, they haven't found a way to turn off the immune attack without using immune-suppressing drugs so potent that they can cause problems as severe as diabetes itself.

Wilkin's idea, the one that made him nearly hit the brake in the middle of the street, sounded ridiculous to the immunologists who first read about it in the pages of *Autoimmunology,* and it still sounds foolish to many diabetes specialists: autoimmune disorders, he proposed, are not really disorders of the immune system. Maybe the organs that the immune system begins attacking actually have something wrong with them, and are sending the standard, appropriate signals to the immune system that all damaged cells have the molecular garbage collectors sweep them away. Maybe the immune attack is really just the smoke, not the fire.

Wilkin's first paper on the subject was published in 1990 under the title "The primary lesion theory of autoimmunity: a speculative hypothesis." By "primary lesion," he meant that something had gone wrong first with the cells or organ, and only afterward had the immune system swooped in for the attack. Instead of autoimmunity being a deadly, counterproductive attack on innocent, healthy cells, he wrote, "autoimmunity is physiologically appropriate and protective. The cell death and tissue damage which results is characteristic of an immune response programmed to eliminate immunogen, remove detritus and isolate the lesion." Put another way, in Wilkin's view, the immune system is just doing its garbage-disposal job of shoveling up tissues that were already diseased, disordered, or dying. He did not, however, apply the idea in that first paper to type 1 diabetes specifically, discussing it only in the broadest possible terms of autoimmune disease generally.

Four years after he first proposed the idea, the editors of the *International Archives of Allergy and Immunology* thought enough of it to publish a pro-and-con pair of articles, with Wilkin taking the pro side and two German researchers taking the con to point out some difficult-to-dispute faults. From there, the hypothesis went through a fallow period. Then, in 1998, after four years of being cocooned in the back of Wilkin's mind, it reemerged, having undergone a metamorphosis. This new version of his hypothesis wasn't about autoimmune diseases in general. This time, it was all about diabetes in particular.

To weave his revised hypothesis, Wilkin stole, magpie-like, from a startling array of seemingly disconnected study findings and emerging trends. First and foremost, of course, was the indisputable fact that both type 1 and type 2 diabetes were rising, seemingly in sync. The orthodox explanations for what causes the two diseases were silent on why this peculiar coincidence should be.

Second: People with type 1 were showing many of the same characteristics as those with type 2, and vice versa. For instance, children and adults with type 1 were now often found to weigh more, on average, than their friends and family members without the disease. In fact, even before they develop type 1, those children destined to do so are heavier as toddlers than their peers who do not. At the same time, people with type 2 diabetes, which supposedly has nothing to do with an autoimmune attack, were sometimes found to have some of the same autoantibodies to the insulin-producing islet cells that only people with type 1 are supposed to have. Studies have found that up to 30 percent of type 2s have the autoantibodies, which makes no sense if obesity is the only cause.

Third: Insulin resistance, the diagnostic hallmark of type 2, could sometimes be detected in children before they develop type 1.

Fourth: Just as type 2 was being seen in younger and younger people, in their twenties and teens, so type 1 was also being seen at younger and younger ages, in an ever-increasing proportion of children under the age of five.

Fifth: The proportion of type 1 diabetics who have the genetic mutations associated with a high risk of developing the disease is getting smaller and smaller, suggesting that genetics is playing a lesser role in the development of diabetes.

Wilkin took these and other facts, shook vigorously, hybridized them with the original hypothesis that had almost brought his car to a stop in the middle of the road, and brought forth what he called the Accelerator Hypothesis.

First set in print in July of 2001 in the eminent European journal *Diabetologia* under the title "The accelerator hypothesis: weight gain as the missing link between type I and type II diabetes," Wilkin laid out the audacious idea that type 1 and type 2 are really one disease, distinguishable only in degrees. A person with a strong genetic tendency to develop diabetes will do so at the drop of a hat, with even a modest increase in childhood weight, and develop what we call type 1. Someone with less of a genetic predisposition will develop it more slowly, requiring more time, more weight, and more insulin resistance, and be labeled as having type 2. The increase in weight, in other words, has *accelerated* the development of diabetes both in those with the greatest inborn genetic risk and those with the least.

To many physicians who treat diabetes, and to many diabetics as well, this idea initially seemed so ridiculous on its face as to be unworthy of serious consideration. *Of course type 1 and type 2 are different,* the skeptics said. *There might be a little overlap, but the vast majority of type 1 diabetics get it early in life, are thin, have no insulin resistance, but do have antibodies against their own beta cells, a sign of an immune attack; whereas the vast majority of type 2 diabetics get it late in life, are fat, have no antibodies, but do have insulin resistance.*

It turned out, however, that the Accelerator Hypothesis would be worthy of a great deal of serious consideration, as evidenced by the five clinical trials that have been conducted so far to test it and the more than 100 papers, for and against, that have cited it in the scientific literature to date. Despite receiving angry public dressings-down at major medical conferences by some of the most prominent researchers in the field, many of whom continue to question his hypothesis in part or whole, Wilkin insists that no serious refutation of it has yet been offered, whether conceptually or experimentally, and that no other compelling hypothesis has been presented to explain the puzzling set of facts of which he has sought to make sense.

MAKING THE CASE

Ironically enough, Wilkin was on the road again when I caught up with him on his cell phone, this time driving across the English countryside with his wife, Linda, herself a PhD who also conducts diabetes research.

"Terry accepts nothing that he is told about anything without questioning it," Linda told me on the speaker phone. Asked whether that could be an occasional annoyance in their home life, she answered diplomatically, "It's a very good virtue."

Why, I asked him, would increased weight make a child or young adult more likely to develop diabetes? Increased weight, he explained, makes the insulin-producing beta cells in the pancreas work harder.

"And when beta cells work harder," he said, "two things happen. First of all they die off quicker, and second, they increase their exposure to the immune system, so that the immune system takes notice of these over-pressured beta cells. What I'm suggesting is that the immune attack is the normal response of the immune system to up-regulated, overloaded beta cells."

At least half a dozen studies from around the world have borne out the relationship between weight and type 1. In Britain, a 2003 study led by Wilkin involving 94 children with type 1 found that the greater their body-mass index, the younger their age of diagnosis.

In Germany and Austria, a 2005 study of 9,248 children with type 1 concluded, "A higher BMI was associated with a younger age at diabetes onset."

In Sweden, a 2008 study concluded, "Rapid growth before seven years of age and increased BMI in childhood are risk factors for later type 1 diabetes. These findings support the accelerator/beta-cell stress hypothesis."

In Australia, a study published in January of 2009 followed 546 children from birth, all of whom had a parent or sibling with type 1 diabetes. By age five and a half, 46 of the children had autoantibodies to their own insulin-producing beta cells, evidence of an immune attack that often results in diabetes. The children's weight and body-mass index, the researchers found, were "continuous predictors of risk of islet autoimmunity," meaning that as weight and BMI went up, so did their risk of early immune attack.

And so on. Not all the studies have been entirely consistent, but in the messy world of human studies, it's now generally accepted that increased childhood weight is associated with an increased risk of type 1. For any individual child, of course, the absolute risk of getting type 1 because of having a few extra pounds is incredibly small. Still, when comparing hundreds or thousands of children, the trend toward increased risk with increased weight is clear and statistically significant. And the relationship, by the way, holds not only for weight and BMI, but also for height. That Swedish study, for instance, found that "children who developed diabetes had experienced more pronounced gain in both weight and height." Altogether, it appears that the faster a child grows, whether up or out, the greater the stress is on the insulin-producing beta cells in the pancreas, and the higher the odds are of developing diabetes.

And it's not just the child's weight that affects his or her risk of developing diabetes — the mother's weight during pregnancy also has an effect, above and beyond any genetic contribution. While in the womb, exposure to a mother's insulin resistance and high levels of weight-related hormones has been shown in repeated studies to increase the developing fetus's risk of growing up to become diabetic. And astonishingly, the same effect has been shown across three generations, so that even the grandfather's childhood diet has an effect on the grandchild's risk of diabetes. Swedish researchers reported in 2002 that people whose grandfathers had lived through a period of famine prior to puberty had one-fourth the risk of developing diabetes as those whose grandfathers had been raised during times of plenty. The accelerating effect of weight, in other words, is transgenerational.

But the Accelerator Hypothesis, Wilkin reminded me, is not just about weight: "The next point is that if you look at children who are not yet diabetic, these children are more insulin resistant than their peers. They have exactly the same physiology as the individual who is going to develop type two. They have high insulin resistance." One of the key studies supporting this view was published in *Diabetologia* in 2004. Researchers at the Walter and Eliza Hall Institute of Medical Research in Melbourne, Australia, examined 104 children, all of whom had autoantibodies to their beta cells, as well as a first-degree relative with type 1. Over a period of four years, 43 of the children progressed to diabetes themselves, while the remainder did not. But at the beginning of the study, years before any of them was actually diabetic, those who would later progress to diabetes had significantly higher insulin resistance compared to those who did not progress. Two other studies have reached the same conclusion, including one from the University of South Florida in Tampa, which concluded, "There is clear evidence of the association between insulin resistance and progression to type 1 diabetes."

The increasing weight of children, Wilkin told me, is not just making type 1 more likely; it's also made the average age of diagnosis increasingly young. "If you look at the epidemiology of type one," he said, "it was always a disease that developed predominantly in a child going through puberty. But in the past ten years, the biggest growth in type one has been in the children under five. The whole thing has shifted—accelerated, I daresay—from adults and adolescents to youth and very small children."

But if type 1 and 2 are really the same disease, I asked him, shouldn't people with type 2 have the same autoantibodies against their beta cells that people with type 1 have? In fact, Wilkin told me, a growing number of studies are showing just that. He pointed to a 2001 study from the Cleveland Clinic Foundation of 101 people with type 2 diabetes, which found that 20 percent had at least one of the autoantibodies normally associated with type 1. Another study published that same year by researchers at the University of Washington of Seattle involved 125 people with recently diagnosed type 2, finding that 29 percent had at least one of the autoantibodies.

After speaking for well over an hour, I thanked the Wilkins for their time and wished them a happy visit with their daughter and soon-to-be-born grandchild. Once I looked over my notes, however, I realized that I was still confused about something. From the time insulin resistance was first identified back in the 1930s, it was always understood to be a problem afflicting the older, heavier diabetics, who needed much more insulin than the younger, thinner diabetics.

Indeed, it's their very need for so much more insulin that justified the term "insulin resistance." So if insulin resistance causes type 1 just as it does type 2, how come the insulin needs of a type 1 are so much less than for a type 2? I emailed Wilkin about my confusion, and he replied: "Start with the basic concept of the Accelerator Hypothesis—tempo. Everybody loses beta cells as part of the ageing process, but for most the loss is not critical in a lifetime. Anything that raises the tempo (accelerates the loss) will result in both earlier presentation and higher incidence (more new cases per year). Insulin resistance is the primary driver of insulin-producing islet cell death, and genes modulate its impact. The probability of diabetes is a combined function of genetic susceptibility and environmental pressure from insulin resistance. If you have high [genetic] susceptibility, relatively little weight or insulin resistance is needed to cause diabetes, and relatively little insulin will be needed to treat it. Lower-risk people will need higher BMI (insulin resistance) to achieve the same probability of developing diabetes, and that tends to be reached later in life. They will also need higher doses of insulin to treat their diabetes."

Put another way, while he believes that type 1 and type 2 are ultimately the same disease, he's not making the patently silly claim that diabetes is the same in everybody. Nor is he saying that it's all caused entirely by weight and weight alone. Rather, a proper understanding of the Accelerator Hypothesis holds that weight simply accelerates the action of two other variables: your genetic tendency to develop insulin resistance in response to weight, and your genetic tendency to have a more or less highly reactive immune system. Imagine, if you will, that your weight, your tendency toward insulin resistance, and your immune reactivity are each ranked on a scale of one to ten. One hundred years ago, only children with the most extreme, hair-trigger immune system, ten out of ten, developed what we think of as type 1 despite being far shorter and skinnier than kids are today. Likewise, only older adults, whose beta cells had been slowly dying off for years due to simple aging, and who had the most extreme tendency toward insulin resistance—ten out of ten—even in the face of only modest weight gains, developed what we now consider to be type 2. Weight, according to the Accelerator Hypothesis, is the enhancer—the MSG, the Special Sauce, if you will—of diabetes risk.

There you have it: a compelling, coherent explanation, supported by a great deal of published evidence, for why diabetes, in both its varieties, has been rising for 150 years, along with body mass. So what's been the reaction of Wilkin's scientific colleagues?

THE CASE AGAINST

"I think it's nonsense," a respected type 1 researcher told me, after insisting that I not publish his name because he knows and respects Wilkin personally. "My opinion is that a common pathway for type 1 and type 2 is definitely not correct. I do not think obesity is a primary trigger of that autoimmune process. Produce one bit of evidence, at this point in time, that weight gain is associated with a triggering of autoimmunity of any patients with type 1. Show me one study." Then, displaying the kind of humility characteristic of many leading scientists, he added, "Wouldn't it be great if I was wrong? None of us wants more than to find out what triggers autoimmunity. If I'm wrong, that would be fantastic."

As a group, researchers who tackle diabetes from the perspective of immunology expressed to me the greatest skepticism toward the Accelerator Hypothesis, perhaps because of its demotion of the immune system as the disease's prime mover. Most of them were willing to concede that weight might play some role in raising the risk of type 1 but scoffed at Wilkin's idea that type 1 and type 2 are just two ends of a single spectrum. For them, types 1 and 2 remain two qualitatively different diseases.

"In terms of the notion that somebody who has type 1 or the autoimmune process caused the disease by becoming obese, I don't think so," said Kevan Herold, MD, a professor of immunology and internal medicine at Yale. But, he added, "I would absolutely agree with that notion that it could be that stressors on beta cells, including possibly obesity, render them as better targets for the immune system to attack."

One of the biggest names in diabetes immunology, George S. Eisenbarth, MD, PhD, told me, "I think there's just not much science behind the hypothesis, is my bias. If you become obese, you will become diabetic sooner. But that's not what Terence Wilkin is trying to say." As executive director of the Barbara Davis Center for Childhood Diabetes and professor of pediatrics, medicine, and immunology at the University of Colorado in Denver, Eisenbarth is credited with proving beyond question, in the mid-1980s, that type 1 is caused by an immune attack. Recent genetic studies, he said, had shown that in siblings of children with type 1 with the highest-risk genetic profile, "their risk of developing diabetes might be as high as 70 to 80 percent. That's not leaving a lot of room for obesity to play much of a role."

Other researchers not as closely involved with immunology, however, took a more nuanced view. "I think it is a very interesting hypothesis," said Johnny Ludvigsson, MD, PhD, a professor of pediatrics at Linköping University in Sweden and one of the best-known diabetes researchers in Europe. "The last fifteen, twenty years, there has been an enormous increase of weight in Swedish children. If you take a group of ten-year-old children, they weigh on average half a kilo [about one pound] heavier than ten-year-olds did the year before. Every year's generation is heavier than the last."

Ludvigsson (who got the name Johnny, despite growing up in Sweden, after his grandmother moved to Chicago) emphasized that weight is probably not the only thing that can press the immune system's attack on the insulin-producing beta cells. "When I talk about beta cell stress," he told me, "I don't want to talk about only weight and insulin resistance. I want to speak broader than that. A lot of different factors stress the beta cells or lead to increased demand for insulin. Even psychological stress can lead to counter-regulatory hormones, which lead to more insulin, and more stress on the beta cells."

Another take came from Jerry P. Palmer, MD, director of the Diabetes Endocrinology Research Center at the University of Washington in Seattle. "I think it's a good idea, and it's a great name," he told me. But, he said, beyond needing more evidence to support all its claims, the hypothesis might make too little of the often glaring differences between type 1 and type 2. "Rather than saying there is just one type of diabetes," he said, "I would go exactly the opposite way, that there might be many types, and we really don't understand all the other causes of beta cell dysfunction."

In fact, some diabetes specialists have proposed that people who have signs of both an autoimmune attack on their beta cells and insulin resistance due to obesity have what they call "double diabetes." One researcher closely associated with this view is Dr. Dorothy Becker, chief of endocrinology and diabetes at Children's Hospital of Pittsburgh. To anyone still clinging to the image of type 1 children being skinny, she said, "You'd better come and visit us. No more. That's where our double diabetes comes from. They're not thin anymore. We've got so many obese kids, we don't know what thin ones look like. If they're not obese at early diagnosis, seventy percent are obese within nine months." For many of her overweight type 1 patients, Becker told me, she now prescribes not only insulin but also metformin, usually considered a drug exclusively for the treatment of type 2.

Even while factors like weight that are normally considered the hallmarks of type 2 are now being seen in type 1, researchers are also finding the converse to be true: a factor once thought to play a role exclusively in type 1—immune dysfunction—has been shown to also play a role in type 2. Three papers published simultaneously in the prominent journal *Nature Medicine* in July of 2009 reported, for the first time, that immune dysfunction in fat cells of overweight people and mice might be the real cause of their diabetes, rather than the fat cells per se. One of the papers even found that two over-the-counter allergy medications, Zaditor and cromolyn, worked better than dietary changes in causing weight loss and relieving diabetes in mice.

What's more, a growing number of adults diagnosed with type 2 have also been shown to have autoantibodies to their beta cells, the precise disorder once thought to affect only people with type 1. Some researchers use the term "type 1.5" to describe such cases. Still others have used the term "latent autoimmune diabetes of adults," or LADA. And then there are those who say this preponderance of names and categories has gotten out of hand, and cannot continue ad absurdum.

This tussle over naming rights has in fact marked the field ever since Himsworth first came up with the distinction, back in 1936, between "insulin-sensitive" and "insulin-insensitive," which then became known as "juvenile" and "adult" diabetes, before morphing into the supposedly more accurate "insulin-dependent diabetes mellitus" or "non-insulin-dependent diabetes mellitus," before doctors finally gave up trying to be descriptive and went with the utterly cryptic "type 1" and "type 2."

THE HALLE BERRY AFFAIR

So confusing has the nomenclature for diabetes become that even many health professionals have become lost, such as the school nurse in Logan, West Virginia, who insisted to me that any of her students taking insulin were, by definition, type 1. And then there is the remarkable case of actress Halle Berry. Back in 1989, she told the British newspaper the *Daily Mail*, "Diabetes caught me completely off guard. None of my family had suffered from the illness and although I was slightly overweight in school, I thought I was pretty healthy. I fell ill—dramatically—when I was on the TV show, *Living Dolls*, in 1989. I felt I needed energy but I didn't even have a minute to pop out and get a chocolate bar. I didn't really know what was wrong. I thought I could tough it out, but I couldn't have been more wrong. One day, I simply passed out, and I didn't wake up for seven days, which is obviously very serious." Her doctors at the hospital, she said, told her that she would need insulin injections for the rest of her life. And as a celebrity spokesperson at the time of the interview for the insulin manufacturer Novo Nordisk, she put a predictably cheerful spin on her need for daily injections. "Actually I feel very lucky that I can take insulin," she said. "It saves me from becoming ill. I have to test my blood sugar levels at least a couple of times a day. I do a tiny pinprick, usually on my fingertips, and test it with a special kit which tell me how high or low my blood sugar levels are. Then using this as a guide I inject myself with the correct dose of insulin to level up my blood sugar."

Reading her account, and seeing her impossibly svelte figure stepping from the surf in an orange bikini in the 2002 James Bond movie *Die Another Day*, one might be forgiven for assuming she must be a type 1. Indeed, the *New York Times* identified her as such in a May 2006 article, as have other media outlets. But then, in an interview with the website contactmusic.com in October of 2007, she was quoted as saying, "I've managed to wean myself off insulin, so now I like to put myself in the type 2 category." She claimed that she had managed the feat through diet and exercise.

She might as well have said that the moon is made of green cheese, to judge by the heated responses from doctors, journalists, and bloggers wedded to the orthodoxy of type 1 versus type 2. For instance, ABC NEWS.com opened its article on the subject with this firm assertion: "Despite her claims to the contrary, Halle Berry did not cure herself of Type 1 diabetes, doctors told ABC NEWS.com, for one simple reason—Type 1 diabetes is incurable." Blogger Kelly Kunik, a type 1 since the age of eight, called Berry's assertion that she had become a type 2 by virtue of weaning herself from insulin "insane" and "moronic."

Such criticisms hold water only if one buys the standard view that type 1 is caused by an autoimmune attack, type 2 by obesity, and never the twain shall meet. But as Wilkin explained to me, "Until the 1990s, we saw the ends of the spectrum, which we interpreted as different diseases. Now we're seeing the ends converge into a single disease." By Wilkin's lights, it makes perfect sense that a young African-American woman who was "slightly overweight in school" should have a form of diabetes that doesn't fit the classic either/or archetypes and might be amenable to diet and exercise. Perhaps she never would have developed it in the first place, or at least not until much later in life, had she not been living in our accelerated era.

One of the most balanced views on Wilkin's hypothesis published so far appeared in *Diabetologia* in a 2007 piece by its editor, Edwin A. M. Gale, MD, of the University of Bristol, in England. "Biological science notoriously leads us into a world of increasing complexity, and concepts that purport to rearrange familiar observations into a new and simpler pattern therefore merit careful consideration," he began. "Such is the accelerator hypothesis, proposed by Terry Wilkin." On the one hand, he called it "brilliantly named and eloquently advocated," yet he also acknowledged that "many have dismissed the arguments out of hand."

After subjecting Wilkin's theory to a brilliant, detailed point-by-point critique, Gale then asked, "Is the accelerator hypothesis therefore beyond salvage? Not entirely. Its strength lies in the fact that accelerators are undoubtedly present." He acknowledged that "children destined to develop type 1 diabetes grow faster and fatter in early life," and that the increase in childhood obesity over the past 50 years "may have contributed to the linear rise of childhood type 1 diabetes." He balanced this by adding that "other accelerators, however, whether genetic, metabolic or immune, are also likely to be present. These, in my view, are fruitful areas for investigation and debate—and could in time lead to the rebirth of the accelerator hypothesis in a new guise."

But what might these other accelerators be? And how strong a role might they be playing in Weston's cluster of ten cases in a two-mile radius in 24 months? Before moving on to the next of the Big Five, I want to give a nod to two other potential accelerators that may be playing a role.

First, Gale himself has studied the effect of mothers' age at delivery. He published a study in *BMJ* (formerly known as the *British Medical*

Journal) in 2000, showing that a mother's risk of giving birth to a child who would later develop type 1 increased by 25 percent for every five years she aged, so that the offspring of a 45-year-old mother has *triple* the risk of developing type 1 as the offspring of a 20-year-old. He also found that each successive child born to a mother has a 15 percent reduced risk of developing diabetes than the sibling born previously, meaning that a populace of large families will tend to have a lower rate of diabetes overall among their children than a populace of smaller families. Altogether, Gale calculated, the rise in Britain's average maternal age in the three decades between 1970 and 2000 caused an 11 percent increase in the incidence of diabetes there. A similar rise in average maternal age in the United States might also be partially behind the rising rate of type 1.

Secondly, and more provocatively, another factor that could be accelerating diabetes risk is, simply put, money. Puzzling though it may be, countless studies have observed that increased wealth translates into increased risk of type 1 — not only within countries (with wealthier people often showing a higher risk), but between countries. For instance, ethnic Finns who live in the western portion of Russia have only one-sixth the risk of developing type 1 as their genetically identical cousins living across the border in Finland. The most striking difference between the two: more money, and a much higher standard of living, in Finland than in Russia. Likewise, as countries have prospered economically, their rates of type 1 have often shot up. As Poland's economy took off along with other parts of Eastern Europe, for example, its annual incidence of type 1 jumped from 4.7 per 100,000 in 1989 to 15.2 per 100,000 in 2002 — more than tripling in just 14 years. Remarkably, studies have also shown that when people from poorer countries immigrate to wealthier ones — say, from Africa to Israel, or from Eastern Europe to Italy — their children's risk of developing type 1 almost instantly becomes as high as their new countries' rate. A 2001 paper in *Diabetologia* even went so far as posing the question in its title, "Is childhood-onset type 1 diabetes a wealth-related disease?" Its answer, based on statistical analysis of rates across Europe, was, "The wide variation in childhood type I diabetes incidence rates within Europe could be partially explained by indicators of national prosperity."

Of course, it can't be that money, in and of itself, is causing the disease. If that were true, the global recession might be the best thing to ever happen to prevent diabetes. More reasonably, it must be something that money buys.

Like milk.

CHAPTER 6

The Cow's Milk Hypothesis

*Does Baby Formula in the First Months of Life
Set off an Immune Attack?*

T HIS STORY ABOUT MOTHER'S milk begins with a bottle of rare
single-malt scotch, which to certain aficionados may sound
redundant. It's the story of a diabetes specialist who knew
little about autoimmunology, an immunologist who knew nothing
and cared less about diabetes, and how the former bribed the latter
with a wee dram into undertaking a study whose findings may soon
permit scientists, for the first time in history, to prevent half or more
cases of type 1.

"He had this absolutely wonderful single-malt scotch," recalled
Hans-Michael Dosch, MD, the immunologist in the story, when I met
him at his laboratory at the University of Toronto's Hospital for Sick
Children—the same institution, by the way, where Drs. Banting and
Best had discovered insulin back in 1922. "You couldn't buy it in a liquor
store. Some friend of his had sent it from Scotland. And oh, it was out
of this world. And I said, 'Julio, I know you; you want something.'"

It was the final Friday of August 1984, and Julio M. Martin, MD,
just a couple of weeks shy of his 62nd birthday, did indeed want
something. He had invited Dosch to drop by his office, as was their

occasional custom, for an end-of-the-week drink and chat. Remarkably friendly, gentle, and humorous, Martin took an old-school physiologist's approach to his diabetes research as senior scientist at the hospital's Research Institute. In the 1970s, he had been the first to show that islet cells, transplanted into diabetic rats, could survive and produce insulin for months. But his and Dosch's lines of research never crossed; they just liked and respected each other, and shared European roots. Dosch was from Marburg, Germany; Martin, although born and raised in Argentina, had maintained close ties to relatives in Switzerland, and had forged collaborations with leading diabetes researchers not only in Scotland but also in Finland, Sweden, and the Netherlands.

Four months earlier, however, Martin had published a trail-blazing study that, if pursued, would bump him right up against Dosch's field. The study had been prompted by a provocative observation made by a friend and colleague from New Zealand, Robert B. Elliott, MD, of the University of Auckland. Elliott had noticed that type 1 diabetes was remarkably rare in Third World countries where the consumption of meat and other proteins was also very low. But when ethnic Chinese moved from Singapore to Australia, their rate of type 1 became equal to that of native Australians, virtually overnight. Likewise, when Polynesian children emigrated from Western Samoa, where type 1 was virtually nonexistent, to Auckland, their rate soared to one out of every 2,000 children—the same as for other New Zealanders. Could it be, the two physicians wondered, that a high-protein diet leads to the development of type 1?

Drs. Elliott and Martin decided to test their diet hypothesis on a strain of non-obese rats who were genetically predisposed to spontaneously develop the equivalent of type 1. From the time of weaning, Martin and Elliott fed 21 of these rats with a low-protein diet. Seven of them received nothing else; seven also received added wheat protein, and the remaining seven, powdered milk. After 133 days, only 15 percent of the rats on the low-protein diet had developed diabetes, compared to 35 percent of those who received additional wheat protein and 52 percent of those supplemented with powdered milk. The results, they concluded in *Diabetologia,* "provide some rationale for speculating that increased dietary intake of protein may be involved in the pathogenesis of the disease in children."

The next logical step was to prove that in diabetes-prone rats, a diet rich in protein from wheat or milk resulted in increased levels of autoantibodies against their own islet cells, sign of an immune attack. Such a study, alas, was beyond Martin's skill set.

On the other hand, it was precisely the kind of technical immunologic work at which Dosch excelled. Then age 37, Dosch had seen his star rise in the late 1970s when he had been on the team that cured one of the "bubble boys" who lacked a properly functioning immune system by transplanting thymus cells, where the immune system's famous "killer T cells" (the T is for thymus) grow, from a donor into a patient. The work had led to important papers on the functioning of T cells in two of the most prominent journals in the world, *Nature* and the *New England Journal of Medicine.*

All of a sudden, Dosch went from being a young, unknown scientist with a poor command of English to having enough of a profile that he was being invited to give lectures at meetings around the world. And now Dr. Martin, with the bottle of rare scotch, was asking him to cast all that aside to pursue a half-baked theory about a possible risk factor for diabetes. "I can't learn all this new-fangled immunology stuff you do," Martin told Dosch, "but I think we need it."

Dosch could spell *diabetes,* but that was about it. He had learned about it in medical school, of course, along with heart disease, hearing loss, and athlete's foot, but understood nothing about it on a serious level. And he had no interest in getting mixed up with it.

Still, for now, all Martin wanted was a little help. A young diabetes researcher was arriving from Finland the very next week on a fellowship. Martin was good friends with this researcher's mentor. The young fellow, Mikael Knip, needed to earn his spurs. Couldn't Dosch see his way to let Knip work in his immunology lab, learn the ropes, and maybe collaborate on a research project?

"What this wonderful bastard did, it's true, he dragged me kicking and screaming into the diabetes realm," Dosch told me. "Julio convinced me I should let Mikael Knip become a fellow in my lab. All of a sudden we had a diabetes project. I helped him a little bit and then I got hooked. I was bushwhacked, and I'm still recovering from it."

MEETING IN ONNELA

The study on which Dosch and Knip collaborated during that year didn't work out. But Knip became comfortable running around an immunology lab, and Dosch got up to speed on diabetes—so much so that five years later, Dosch was invited to join Martin, Knip, and a few other leading diabetes researchers from around the world for an exclusive brainstorming session at the summer cottage of Knip's mentor in Janakkala, Finland. Only it wasn't summer. The group arrived at the home, located in the countryside less than 300 miles south of the Arctic Circle, on January 10, 1989. The next morning, the sun crawled over the horizon around 9:30 A.M., spent six hours casting a feeble twilight, and then slipped back into the netherworld shortly after 3 P.M. A storm snowed in the group of seven, but nobody minded. The house was named Onnela, which means "happiness," and the group happily hunkered down.

Their host was Hans K. Åkerblom, MD, professor and chairman of pediatrics at the University of Helsinki's Hospital for Children and Adolescents. Himself a type 1 since the age of 14, in 1949, Åkerblom had devoted his career to his fellow diabetics. During the 1960s, he had focused on improving the treatment of children with the disease. In the 1970s he had grown interested in epidemiology, particularly the question of why Finland, then as now, should have the highest rate of type 1 diabetes in the world. By the 1980s he had turned his attention to etiology, the pathogenesis of the disease, and what if anything might be done to nip it in the bud.

Four lines of evidence had convinced Åkerblom and his six guests that they weren't insane for imagining that prevention might be possible:

- First was the 1984 study by Martin and Elliott, both now among the invited guests, showing that wheat protein increased the rate at which rats developed type 1, and cow's milk increased it even more.

- Second, a study published that very month in *Diabetologia* confirmed findings in the United States and elsewhere that breastfed infants have a lower risk of later developing type 1 than those who had received formula.

- Third, Åkerblom and his colleagues had recently discovered that children with type 1 had significantly higher levels of antibodies to cow's milk protein than did children without the disease.

- And fourth, international variations in per-capita consumption of milk correlated well with the incidence rates for type 1. Finns, for instance, drank more milk than citizens of any other country, an average of 48 gallons per year for every man, woman, and child; and their risk of developing type 1, as noted above, was also the highest in the world. The Chinese, on the other hand, who enjoyed one of the lowest levels of type 1 in the world, drank on average just 2.3 gallons of milk per year.

"I was convinced that cow's milk is a culprit," Åkerblom told me when reached by telephone in Helsinki, where he is now professor emeritus and confined to a wheelchair due to severe osteoporosis, but otherwise in reasonable health after 60 years with type 1. Much as he believed in the cow's milk hypothesis, however, he invited the other researchers there to pick it apart, see if it could hold up to critique, and, if it did, plot a course of action.

"Julio Martin was one of the first to have the hypothesis," Åkerblom said. "So I invited him, as well as Dr. Elliott from New Zealand. Then we had Professor Allan Drash from the University of Pittsburgh, and Franco Botazzo from Italy." Botazzo, back in 1974, had been the first to report the presence of antibodies to islet cells in the blood of type 1 diabetics. Dosch and Knip rounded out the group.

"We got to really discuss and talk in great depth, because we were stuck there for days," Dosch told me. "It was dark all day. We were having a good time. By the end of that week, we had some sort of road map of what we were going to do about type one diabetes. There was a very specific moment when we all came to the same conclusion, that if there was any truth to what we were thinking, we might be able to prevent diabetes. Today scientists are talking all the time about diabetes prevention. But in 1989, it was almost blasphemy. The thought of that time was, 'You got diabetes, too bad. We'll never be able to do anything about it.'"

Everyone agreed that the only way to ultimately prove or disprove the hypothesis was with a randomized clinical trial, with infants getting either a cow's milk formula or not, to see what effect it had on their risk of developing type 1 diabetes. But such a study would be extraordinarily complex, lengthy, and expensive, and they hadn't yet laid the groundwork. To silence the skeptics who would surely question the need for mounting a large clinical trial, they had to first put together an airtight case for a mechanism showing how cow's milk protein fosters an immune attack that results in diabetes years later. To which of the dozens of different proteins in cow's milk did the human immune system react? During what period in infancy does the immune reaction occur? Which components of our immune system mount the attack?

To answer these complex questions, the natural point man was the one researcher in the room who had never before published a

The Cow's Milk Hypothesis

study of diabetes, but who just happened to be a master of cutting-edge immunology.

RIDER ON THE STORM

"I am a risk taker," Dosch said.

He stood on the balcony of his apartment high above the shore of Lake Ontario, smoking a pipe, drinking a bottle of Warsteiner Premium Verum, a beer popular in his native Germany, and gazing at the spot where he had capsized his sailboat within view of the shoreline during a terrific storm 15 years earlier.

"I was not with my crew, but with some friends, one an older gentleman," he told me. "He was then as old as I am now," which is 61, "and his girlfriend had never been on a sailboat. We left from my yacht club, right below here. Not a cloud in the sky. Then we saw the weather coming in. I said, 'Ah, I've been sailing here for over twenty years; it's okay.' Eventually we had to take the sails down, it was wild. I'll never forget. This woman, I knew her a little bit, she asks, 'Do these boats capsize? I can't swim.' 'Don't worry,' I say, 'these boats never capsize; they never sink.' A J/24, it's a good boat.

"We got hit by this squall from the side, we were doing 14.5 knots, no sails up; we capsized. I was fortunate this girl was not given to panic. Then a second wave came after that. Since we had no sail, it was easy to turn it upside down. The poor thing toggles. I still wasn't worried. It was warm.

"My friend got tangled, though, as it toggled. I had to swim underneath and help him get out of that. None of us were wearing life vests. These big flaps were unsecured. We then right the boat. These flaps open. Scoops up the bottom, the water was at the level of the deck, and then she sank. She's still down there, poor thing. We were picked up; everyone was fine. I learned a lot, but I lost my boat. In boating, one little thing leads to the next. But I am a risk taker." And with that, he flipped the subject back to his work. "Some people want to move forward bit by bit in science. That would bore me."

Having co-authored 81 studies in the 22 years since the beginning of his career in 1969, Dosch published his first on diabetes in October of 1991. In it, he, Martin, and colleagues reported tantalizing evidence that the same antibodies that react to cow's milk protein in diabetic children also reacted to a protein on the surface of the beta cells. That study, however, was just a warm-up for the main event. In the July 30, 1992, edition of the *New England Journal of Medicine,* Dosch served as senior author of a paper on which Knip, Åkerblom, Martin, and four other colleagues collaborated. The paper began by noting recent studies in animals suggesting that bovine serum albumin, or BSA, is the protein in cow's milk responsible for triggering an auto-immune response, in particular a region on the albumin molecule called ABBOS.

To see if the findings held true in humans, they conducted advanced immunologic tests on the blood serum of 142 children with diabetes, 79 healthy children, and 300 adult blood donors. All the children with diabetes, they found, had high levels of antibodies to the albumin in cow's milk, most of which were specific to ABBOS, whereas only 2.5 percent of the healthy children had ABBOS-specific antibodies.

To judge by the media response, Dosch's risky decision to jump into diabetes research in mid-career had paid off. Among the dozens of news reports around the world that appeared on the day of the study's publication was one in the *New York Times,* quoting him as saying: "Based on our results, we think it's too early to make any general recommendations about avoiding cow's milk without further study. But you are safe in recommending breast feeding for as long as possible before going to formula because studies clearly show that breast feeding reduces the risk of developing diabetes two to three fold in those disposed to the disease." By six to eight months, he said, most children's immune systems and intestinal tract would be sufficiently matured to permit the safe ingestion of cow's milk.

If the press embraced the news, however, most of the U.S. diabetes research establishment did not. The reaction seemed to be, *"Milk? Are you kidding me?"* George Eisenbarth—who was the same age as Dosch, and had attended the same fellowship program in immunology—was by now the reigning star of research into diabetic autoimmunity, and he pronounced the ABBOS findings to be as sour as curdled milk.

A more serious attack came in December of 1993, when Mark Atkinson, PhD, a well-known and well-funded diabetes researcher at the University of Florida College of Medicine in Gainesville, published a follow-up study in the *New England Journal of Medicine.* Atkinson reported that he could find antibodies to cow's milk albumin in general, and to ABBOS in particular, in only two of 24 children who had recently developed type 1, despite the fact that Dosch had given him technical advice and supplied him with the ABBOS peptide. In the history of science, such a challenge could mean only one of three things: Dosch was so skilled in his laboratory techniques that another prominent researcher couldn't reproduce them, or he was so unskilled that he had been unintentionally fooled by his own lousy data—or it was something much worse, the kind of thing that ends a career in shame.

Dosch and colleagues fired back with a letter to the *New England Journal of Medicine,* noting two new studies confirming their results and suggesting that "technical aspects" of Atkinson's work may have contributed to his failure to find the antibodies. That set off the scientific equivalent of a schoolyard rumble, with Atkinson and his colleagues responding, "We believe the statements by Dosch et al. about our ability to detect BSA antibodies are unfounded."

Both sides came away from the fight satisfied that they had retained their honor, done their duty, and were no worse for wear. As other teams around the world confirmed the presence of antibodies to cow's milk proteins, Dosch's finding was accepted as essentially accurate. As for Atkinson, he told me in a telephone interview from his office in Gainesville, where he remains a well-respected scientist, "Part of the story was their assertion that one hundred percent of people with type one make anti-BSA antibodies. Clearly that was errant. The other notion, of early feeding, is still subject to trial and controversy."

Indeed, even as more studies from around the world confirmed it, the cow's milk hypothesis appeared to be the Rodney Dangerfield of theories, getting little respect at major scientific meetings in the United States—perhaps because no U.S. researchers had been directly involved in the original breakthrough paper in the *New England Journal of Medicine*, perhaps because nobody had ever heard of Dosch, or perhaps because the whole theory seemed too pat, too easy.

"I have often wondered why it is so," Åkerblom told me. "Some of those who are well-known scientists, they kept criticizing when we presented at meetings. I don't know if it would just be scientific envy of what we were doing. It was an interesting psychological phenomenon. But some of these strong opponents have changed their opinions over the years. And still we haven't given up."

Indeed, their work to pursue the cow's milk hypothesis was only just beginning. But the next, most important, phase would have to proceed without the benefit of the senior physician who had set the whole process in motion with a bottle of single-malt scotch. Having spent his career investigating the mysteries of the pancreas, Julio Martin died on December 1, 1993, after a long struggle with pancreatic cancer.

ALIEN INVADERS

Having watched the sun set spectacularly from his balcony, Dosch and I went to dinner at the restaurant in his building, accompanied by his beautiful, younger, Portuguese wife, Ana, and their two sons. Twelve-year-old Daniel did his homework at the table, baby Andrew struggled to escape from his high chair, and the restaurant's German owner, a good friend of Dosch's, kept our wineglasses full. With thinning hair fading from blond to white, Dosch reminded me of the late comedic actor Phil Hartman, although with a larger, rounder nose. He wore a tan jacket and supple, brown Italian-style loafers. He had remarkably smooth hands and perfect fingernails, and every once in a while, as he spoke, he would gaze off into the distance and smile, as if glimpsing something stunning.

"Type one diabetes is still mostly a Western disease, but that's changing along with milk consumption," he told me. "You look at Puerto Rico, they now have a huge type one incidence for an Hispanic country. They have this program, WIC [the Special Supplemental Nutrition Program for Women, Infants and Children, administered by the U.S. Department of Agriculture]. It's wonderful, but it has its drawbacks. In Puerto Rico, close to one hundred percent of babies go into the WIC program, which provides free formula, so all of them are on it. The breastfeeding rate in Puerto Rico is like five percent.

"In China, they used to have maybe two cases a year of type one reported, in a country of over a billion people. Now they're hovering around one or two per hundred thousand. That's a major increase. That's twenty thousand new cases per year. That's a lot of diabetics. With this current scandal of melamine in the baby formula, no such thing was even possible until lately. You couldn't get formula in China. They had rice gruel, where they cooked rice for a long time, and they add a little honey. It's a complex carbohydrate. It's not much of an immune challenge."

What is it about milk, I asked him, that does challenge the immune system?

"Cow's milk has a major difference from human milk," he said. "With cow's milk, the major component is casein. You like that because it allows you to make cheese. Human milk has much less, tenfold less casein. If you put a baby on pure cow's milk, particularly early in life, the results aren't very nice. The baby will get colic, because casein is hard to digest; it's a real tough molecule. However, if you change the ratio between casein and the other proteins, and make it more human-like, it becomes much, much easier. So modern formulas make some dramatic changes to the milk."

But, he explained, even if the stomach isn't upset, the immune system often is.

"When you are a newborn, and you are taking in mom's milk, you are basically living in an immunologic universe that is very calm and gentle," he said. "Everything in the body is known to the immune system. And then comes this day, let's say Thursday afternoon, when mom's breasts are inflamed, she's tired, and she says, 'I've had it with this breastfeeding,' and you get your first bottle feeding. And this first feeding in the Western world is almost always a formula based on cow's milk. That's why cow's milk is getting the bad name. If the first food were, say, herring extract, to say something ridiculous, it would have the same effect."

Now I was confused. Isn't this the cow's milk hypothesis? As he explained, yes, it had started out as the cow's milk hypothesis, but studies published in the years since their first papers were published had shown that foreign protein—any foreign protein—has more or less the same effect as cow's milk on a baby's developing immune system when given before six months of age.

"I should make this really clear," Dosch said. "The diabetes risk that comes from early nutrition reflects exposure to complex foreign proteins. If you would try giving giraffe milk to a three-month-old, chances are it would have the same diabetogenic potential. Soy milk will do it too. Someone once asked about donkey milk, but that would also have the same effect, I think.

"The thing is, this baby's immune system has been invaded, overwhelmed, by millions of things it must consider invasive bugs, aliens, literally. It's a serious insult. And if this happens at six months old, it's okay. The immune system has grown up; it has seen maybe bits and pieces of these proteins already. But if it happens well before six months, poof, it's like World War Three for your immune system. In a host that is prone to develop diabetes, the stage has been set. It makes the immune system more permissive toward autoimmunity."

So it could just as well be called the donkey's milk hypothesis?

"Not a whole lot of people will get donkey milk," Dosch said. "It's virtually uniform that when an infant gets formula, it's cow's milk. It's given the cows a bad name, but there you have it."

Indeed, as Julio Martin's first study on the subject showed in 1984, wheat protein can also raise the risk of diabetes. Wheat gluten, in particular, has since been linked not only to type 1 diabetes but also to celiac disease, a disorder in which the intestines become inflamed and damaged in response to gluten. This may explain why the two disorders often appear together in the same individuals.

In fact, many of the genes that have been associated with type 1 appear to act on neither the immune system nor the pancreas, but on the permeability of the gut. So-called "leaky" guts apparently permit these foreign proteins to creep into the pancreatic lymph nodes, where killer T cells see them and begin ramping up the attack that will end up destroying the insulin-producing beta cells (or, in the case of celiac disease, the intestines). Milk protein, wheat protein, herring extract—to the infant immune system in the first six months of life, they're all just Mongol hordes.

The part about wheat protein is particularly ironic, however, considering that Toronto's Hospital for Sick Children, where insulin was discovered, Martin worked, and Dosch remains, was also the place where pediatricians invented Pablum, the first dried, precooked baby food, which to this day includes wheat. In its first 25 years on the market, beginning in 1931, the hospital received a royalty on every package of Pablum sold. As Dosch put it, "This hospital was built on Pablum money."

But Pablum was hardly the first prepared baby food to be sold. That distinction goes to Soluble Food for Babies, which went on sale all the way back in 1867—just around the time, it should be noted, that rates of both type 1 and 2 began their historic ascent. While most infants were still breastfed at the beginning of the 20th century, by the early 1960s fully 90 percent were on the bottle. True, breastfeeding has been paid a great deal of, um, lip service since then. But a study published in the *Archives of Pediatrics and Adolescent Medicine* noted in September of 2008 that "exclusive breastfeeding rates among young infants are discouragingly low," with a mere 11 percent of U.S. infants exclusively breastfed at six months of age. Despite a wealth of data establishing the benefits of exclusive breastfeeding, the study found that most U.S. hospitals on the East Coast give away free samples of formula to new mothers. "The commercial sample packs contain formula, coupons, advertisements and baby products," the study found. The giveaways, they noted, "have been shown to undermine breastfeeding, and their elimination from U.S. hospitals may help to increase exclusive breastfeeding rates nationally."

With the vast majority of infants still receiving at least some supplemental feedings before six months of age despite decades of ferocious advocacy by pediatricians and other health groups, what possible hope could there be for Dosch, Knip, Åkerblom, and others to convince them to stop giving formula to babies in order to prevent type 1 diabetes?

TRIGR

Luckily, that's not something the researchers have to worry about. As it happens, giving up all bottle feeding is unnecessary; all that has to be eliminated from the infants' diet are the large, naturally occurring protein chains that the immune system recognizes as foreign. "Basically the protein has to be split into such small fragments that the immune system can't see it," Dosch explained to me. "And still it has the same nutritional value as the natural protein. It's called highly hydrolyzed formula. You can pick it up in any drugstore. It was developed for infants with allergies to cow's milk. It's been around for like fifty years."

Once Dosch's initial findings were published in the *New England Journal of Medicine* in 1992, the original cadre of conspirators from Åkerblom's cottage immediately set to work to begin testing what would happen if they randomized infants to receive either a standard milk formula or one that was highly hydrolyzed, or fragmented.

"The main question at first was to find out: is it feasible to get mothers to take part in such a thing?" Åkerblom said. "Beginning our first pilot study here in 1992, we found twenty agreeing mothers. So we knew it was at least feasible. We did a second larger study of two hundred forty children, beginning in nineteen ninety-five. This was expanded to Finland, Sweden, and Estonia."

Working with infants who had a first-degree relative previously diagnosed with type 1 diabetes and displaying autoimmune markers, they encouraged mothers to breastfeed if possible but supplied them with formula, either standard or highly hydrolyzed, if they chose to supplement their infant's diet. In 2008, Knip reported that in the study of 240 children, their risk of either developing type 1 or having two autoantibodies to the insulin-producing beta cells in the pancreas was cut by well over half in those who had been fed highly hydrolyzed formula, compared to those who had been normally fed with standard formula.

By then, though, the group had already moved on to the final study they had dreamed up 19 years earlier, a stunningly ambitious and costly one designed to nail down the truth (or not) of the cow's milk (for lack of a better term) hypothesis once and for all: the Trial to Reduce IDDM (Insulin Dependent Diabetes Mellitus) in the Genetically at Risk, or TRIGR. Beginning in May of 2002, 76 medical centers from 15 countries in Europe, Australia, and North America began recruiting participants for the study.

"We have now more than 2,160 children in follow-up," Åkerblom said. By the time all the children have reached age six, he said, it will be the autumn of 2012. Only then will the TRIGR group "un-blind" their data to see which children received the highly hydrolyzed formula as infants and which received the standard. At that point, they will be able to announce whether or not it made a difference in their risk of having markers of an immune attack underway. Not for another four years later, when all the children turn ten, will they know if it made a difference on the bottom line: progression to actual diabetes.

"I'm expecting it to prevent close to eighty percent of cases of type one," Dosch told me.

Åkerblom wasn't so sure. "I would be more careful in putting a percentage on it," he said. "Our study protocol is based on being able to detect a forty to fifty percent effect. That may be pushing it. I wouldn't put it to eighty. There are so many factors in human life in children."

What if, I asked him, the study finds no significant effect either way after all their work?

"Nothing is certain," he replied. "But if that would be the case, it would still be important to know, because then we would not have to worry about cow's milk in children. If it's positive, there are clearly consequences. But whatever the results, it is scientifically important. Until then, the hypothesis is still debatable. Many, many scientists are critical and doubtful. I am confident that the result will be valuable."

In the meanwhile, I asked Åkerblom, would it be prudent for parents who have type 1 diabetes themselves, or already have a child with it, to use only highly hydrolyzed formula in the event that they do not exclusively breastfeed? (Frankly, I was thinking of the people in Weston, and towns like it, where parents are alarmed about the rising rate of type 1 and eager to try something simple to prevent it.)

"No, we have not yet proven it scientifically," he said. "My advice would be to follow the normal feeding routes before we have the results available. We have had a strong emphasis in our study group not to start giving premature infant nutrition guidance before we know more about the results."

And what if he does not live to see the results? By 2012, after all, he will be close to 80.

"I am happy every day I am still around," Åkerblom said. "At this age, one cannot be sure if you will be around long enough to see things happen. I am just sitting around these days and writing a history of the TRIGR project. That's what I have been involved in for several months. I'm happy every day I'm still staying alive in a work-about condition."

Of course, that's all good and fine for Åkerblom, but as for me, when my own daughter was a newborn and my wife chose to begin supplementing her feedings, I made sure we bought the highly hydrolyzed formula. It cost a bit more, but from my perspective, it was well worth it.

As for Dosch, although he is serving as leader of Toronto's TRIGR site, he remains ever the risk taker, having lately switched into the university's neurology section to pursue some curious findings. Type 1, he now believes, is really caused by dysfunctioning pain receptors around the pancreas, which set off the alarms that the immune system responds to. Type 2, on the other hand, may really be an autoimmune disorder, just like type 1; he's even shown in obese, diabetic mice that a drug suppressing their immune system also reverses their diabetes. Neurologists, immunologists, and endocrinologists aren't sure what to make of his new work; the only thing certain is that, once again, he has turned conventional wisdom on its head.

Which, one suspects, is just where Dosch likes it.

CHAPTER 7

The POP Hypothesis

The Risks of Persistent Organic Pollutants

YOUR CHILD WITH TYPE 1 is rail thin, you say, and you exclusively breastfed him until he was seven months old? Hang on. Just because weight and baby formula might increase a person's risk of developing diabetes doesn't mean they're the only accelerators of risk.

Some of the other factors being investigated by researchers fall into the variety more typically associated with health scares: manmade environmental toxins. And what better place to begin examining this subject than in Woburn, Massachusetts, the middle-class town just a half-hour drive from its wealthier neighbor Weston? Woburn became nationally known as the setting for *A Civil Action,* the 1996 book by Jonathan Harr and the subsequent movie starring John Travolta. Leukemia diagnosed in over two dozen kids there was linked to the industrial chemicals trichloroethylene (or TCE, widely used as a solvent) and perchloroethylene (or PCE, used for dry-cleaning clothing and degreasing machinery). The chemicals were found at levels 20 to 50 times the safe limit in two municipal wells. Lengthy lawsuits against the firms charged with dumping the chemicals resulted in settlements of just $9 million, even though the Environmental Protection Agency later designated five properties in town to be Superfund sites under the federal program that manages and funds costly cleanups.

Greg and Kristin Ahearn, longtime residents of Woburn, invited me to their home to discuss their theories for why both of their sons, and an unsettling number of their sons' classmates, had recently developed type 1 diabetes.

"Did you talk about the cancer water?" Greg asked Kris when he arrived home from his job as a construction supervisor.

"We weren't ever able to drink the water in my house," Kris said. "It smelled. Growing up, my mother had breast cancer, my neighbor across the street had breast cancer. My aunt had breast cancer. My father's father had stomach cancer; he grew up over there too. Two neighbors had brain tumors. My good friend at the time had leukemia, a boy in second grade. Four of the boys who died of leukemia—Jarrod Aufiero, Michael Zona, Patrick Toomey, Jimmy Anderson—they all lived right in my neighborhood. We were having Ronald McDonald carnivals all the time for these kids. That's what you did, because everybody had it.

"My father's best friend was Tom Mernin, the city engineer. He kept telling my parents, 'There's nothing wrong with that water, I drink it myself.' He died of leukemia in his fifties. My father remembers him holding it in a jar. 'It's perfectly healthy; drink it.'"

Despite the fear of growing up amid such circumstances, Kris felt, until five years ago, that she had dodged a bullet. "It's kind of one of those, you think, 'Wow, I escaped that, it's pretty good.'" Her voice broke, and she blinked her eyes. "My brother and I are okay; my parents are okay now. Then you feel unlucky that your child gets diabetes, and then that both do. You wonder, did I do something?"

Greg, beefy and blue-eyed, squeezed the hand of his pretty, blond wife, who looks younger than her 42 years. The couple and their two sons still live in Woburn, a short drive from the neighborhood where Kris grew up.

"We always wonder if there's a tie," he said. "I think there might be a tie, through the parents who didn't get cancer. There's definitely a possible tie. They tell you they don't know what causes it. Something triggers diabetes and they don't know what. Some event."

"It's frustrating," Kris said. "You have your healthy pregnancy; you do everything you're supposed to do. So what happened? What went wrong?"

THE GOODYEAR SCHOOL

Their older son, Kyle, was in fifth grade at Goodyear Elementary School when, early in January of 2003, he began urinating frequently and drinking a lot of water. Then one night Kris heard him going . . . and going . . . and going. She thought, "That's just not normal."

The next day, Kyle had baseball camp. He wasn't feeling well but went anyway. When Greg brought him home, he told Kris, "What a waste of money, he's not even swinging the bat at this camp."

Kyle broke into tears. "I'm too tired to swing the bat," he said, "and I can't see the ball anyway."

Something went off in Kris's mind; she put the puzzle together. Wiping up the urine on the floor beneath the toilet, she recalled, it had a sticky consistency. She didn't know much about diabetes, except from a cousin whose son had it. Still, the next morning, on Martin Luther King Jr. Day, she called her pediatrician's office at 9:00 and told him, "I think Kyle has diabetes." After she listed his symptoms, the doctor told her she had to bring him over right away. "I'm going to take a shower and get myself together," Kris said.

"No, you need to come right over," said the doctor, apparently concerned that Kyle's blood-sugar level was dangerously high.

When they got there, Kyle's blood sugar turned out to be in the upper 600s, approaching the level that could put a person into a coma. By the time they made it to Massachusetts General Hospital, it had climbed into the 700s, above the level the emergency room's hand-held meter was equipped to measure.

Two days later, Kyle was back in school, where he learned that another boy also had type 1 diabetes. After getting over the initial shock, the family took it more or less in stride, until May of 2004—barely a year after Kyle had been diagnosed—when Kris smelled that fruity, funky scent of rotten apples on the breath of Kyle's eight-year-old brother, Ethan.

"Oh my God, I can smell it, he's got it," Kris told Greg.

"You're always thinking the worst," he said. "He doesn't have it."

The next morning she tested Ethan with Kyle's meter; his blood-sugar level was 275. They went to the pediatrician, who sent them to the hospital to get Ethan's blood sugar back down to earth with his first injections of insulin. Back at Mass General, the pediatric endocrinologist who had diagnosed Kyle couldn't believe they were back with Ethan; the odds of two brothers both getting the disease is only about 6 percent. (Even if type 1 diabetes is diagnosed in an identical twin, the sibling with the identical genes has even odds of never getting the disease—obvious proof that something in the environment or diet must play an important role.)

The next month, Kris heard that seven-year-old Tyler Brinkley, a classmate of Ethan's at Goodyear, was newly diagnosed with type 1 diabetes. The boys both played hockey and ran in the same circles. Two months later, in August, Tyler's five-year-old brother, Christian, was also diagnosed. That same month, another Goodyear student, nine-year-old Nick Cromer, was also diagnosed. Along with another child who had developed type 1 before beginning school, that made seven current or former students with type 1 in a school of 231 students.

According to SEARCH, the ongoing survey of type 1 diabetes being conducted by the CDC in six communities around the country, the average proportion of children ages 17 and under who have type 1 at any given time is currently about 0.5 percent, or one-half of 1 percent. That would mean that the expected number of children with type 1 at the Goodyear school would be one, or maybe two. Not seven.

Early in the summer of 2004, at the urging of parents, Mayor John C. Curran requested that the state's Department of Public Health conduct an investigation. "There is some concern," he told the *Boston Globe*. Initial fears centered around conditions at the 77-year-old Goodyear Elementary School, which contained some mold. But the state investigation found that three of the Goodyear students who developed diabetes had family members with it, and that others were diagnosed years apart. What's more, with a total of 16 type 1 diabetics in all of its public schools, Woburn's overall rate fell well within statistical expectations. Yet since the state report was published in September of 2004, the diagnoses of type 1 have continued piling up.

"In seventh, a girl name Kara got it," said Kyle, sitting with his parents in their living room; at 16, Kyle has been living with his diabetes for six years. "In sixth, two boys got it. Last year, there were two twins."

In the summer of 2008, Ethan, by then 13, had what Kris called a "fling" with another type 1, a girl named Lizzy. Did they ever talk about having the same disease, or did they ever inject at the time? No, answered the shy young man.

"Everybody who got it over at Goodyear, all their parents except one were linked to east Woburn," said Greg, referring to the part of town where Kris had grown up. "Either the mother or father. Then we found out a couple kids in another school had it; their parents grew up in east Woburn too."

"I used to be the mayor's secretary," said Kris. "I had access to all these people. I was just saying, 'You know this is really strange, my second son ended up with diabetes.' Everyone had this overwhelming fear that Woburn was going to get put back on the map with another bad thing attached to it. "They were willing to look into it, but they didn't want to get any press. Not that you can blame them. People still say, 'You live in Woburn? Isn't that where everyone is glowing?'"

Cheryl Beasley, another Woburn native, grew up just around the corner from Kris's childhood home and still lives there. Cheryl's daughter, Kelsey, developed type 1 the same year as Ethan, in 2004. "I know that just within my neighborhood, there's five diabetics," Cheryl told me. "My father died in 'eighty-four of lymphoma. My mother just passed away last year of cancer. I'm sure we all drank the water from those wells. My mother cooked with it."

Tammie Brinkley, another Woburn resident with whom Cheryl grew up, also still lives in the neighborhood. Although two of her sons developed type 1 in 2004, her third boy remains free of the disease.

"I do know we live where the 'Civil Action' water problem was," Tammie said. "I was not satisfied with the report we got from the state. It didn't tell much."

Indeed, the only testing recommended in the state's 2004 report was of Goodyear's indoor air quality, to check for mold and other allergens. It made no reference to the town's history with TCE and PCE in the drinking water, or, for that matter, to any man-made contaminants. And why would it? After all, the contaminated wells were shut down some two decades before any of the children who developed diabetes were born. Surely nature would not be so cruel as to hold the exposures of the mothers and fathers against their children?

TCE, PCE, PCB, ETC.

Back in 1973, Arizona physicians observed that a surprising one-third of all patients with congenital heart disease had grown up in a small area in the Tucson Valley—the same area where groundwater was later found, in 1981, to be contaminated with TCE, and to a lesser extent with another toxic industrial chemical, dichloroethylene, and traces of the metal chromium. As soon as the contamination was discovered, wells in the area were closed, giving researchers the chance to investigate whether any adverse health effects were seen in children born later, who had never been directly exposed to the contaminants themselves but whose parents had. Sure enough, they found that such children had triple the risk of being born with congenital heart defects, compared to children born of parents who had never lived in the contaminated area.

The results of other studies have been mixed. Some have found no birth defects in offspring of trichloroethylene-exposed parents. Others have. For instance, a 2004 study in the journal *Birth Defects Research* found that mothers who were over the age of 38 when they gave birth and had lived within 1.3 miles of a site contaminated with trichloroethylene were six times more likely to give birth to a child with a congenital heart defect compared to mothers who were younger and did not live near a contaminated site.

Whether parents' exposure to trichloroethylene would increase their children's risk of developing type 1 diabetes later in life is entirely unknown; no study on the question has ever been published. But the chemical has been shown to increase blood-sugar levels in humans and animals directly exposed to it. For instance, a review of the published literature on TCE by the Agency for Toxic Substances and Disease Registry (an arm of the Centers for Disease Control) noted in 1995 that diabetes was among the nine diseases associated with it. In its national database, the agency found an increased risk of diabetes in women ages 18 to 24 and 45 to 54 who were exposed to trichloroethylene, but not in women of any other age.

More broadly, growing numbers of studies have found an increased risk of type 2 diabetes in people exposed to a wide variety of industrial contaminants. U.S. Air Force veterans returning from Vietnam after exposure to Agent Orange, which they sprayed on jungles to kill foliage, were one of the first groups in which the effect was seen. The compound contained the herbicide dioxin, later linked to central nervous system damage, thyroid disorders, immune system dysfunction, and diabetes. Air Force investigators reported in 1997 that veterans who participated in spraying Agent Orange were more than twice as likely to be taking oral medications for diabetes as were Air Force veterans who had gone to Vietnam but had not participated in the spraying. A follow-up study, published in 2008 by epidemiologists at the University of Texas Health Science Center in San Antonio, found that the risk of diabetes grew even stronger when they accounted for how many days the veterans had actually spent spraying.

Similar associations have been found in people around the world. In Taiwan, a manufacturing accident resulted in thousands of people in the 1970s consuming rice-bran oil containing high doses of the industrial chemicals known as polychlorinated biphenyls (PCBs) and polychlorinated dibenzofurans (PCDFs). They developed what was called Yu-Cheng (Chinese for "oil disease"), which caused severe toxic reactions. In 2008, researchers at Taiwan's National Health Research Institutes reported that female Yu-Cheng survivors (but not male) were twice as likely to develop type 2 diabetes as women not exposed to the contaminated rice-bran oil. Women who had developed a severe acne-like reaction to the exposure were over five times more likely to develop type 2 diabetes than those who did not have such a reaction.

In Seveso, Italy, a pesticide plant exploded in 1976, exposing thousands of nearby residents to highly toxic doses of dioxin. Up to 25 years later, women who had lived in the vicinity of the plant at the time of the accident (but, again, not the men) were at greater risk of developing type 2 diabetes than were those who lived outside the area.

In Anniston, Alabama, a large plant manufactured PCBs from 1929 to 1971, and contamination remains widespread in the area. On April Fool's Day of 2008, researchers hired by the Agency for Toxic Substances and Disease Registry reported their preliminary conclusions about local health effects of the PCBs at a town meeting in Anniston. "Our findings indicate that levels of PCBs higher than the U.S. average were associated with a two- to four-fold greater prevalence of diabetes in Anniston men and women between the ages of 35 to 54 regardless of obesity, family history, gender, or race," announced study leader Allen Silverstone, PhD, of the State University of New York in Syracuse.

Along the St. Lawrence River that separates New York State from Canada, the Mohawk Nation at Akwesasne maintained its traditional practice of fishing from the river after aluminum foundries contaminated it with PCBs. In 2007, researchers at the University of Albany reported that Native Americans on the reservation with the highest levels of PCB in their blood had almost *four times* the risk of type 2 diabetes of those with the lowest PCB levels.

In New York State overall, another study by the same group at the University of Albany reported in 2007 that residents living in zip codes containing hazardous waste sites were 25 percent more likely to have been hospitalized with a diagnosis of diabetes than were people living outside such sites. That figure held even after the researchers statistically adjusted to account for the possible distorting effects of socioeconomic and other variables. And when they looked just along the Hudson River, where there is higher income, less smoking, better diet, and more exercise than in the state overall, those living near a waste site containing "persistent organic pollutants" (such as dioxin) had a 36 percent higher risk of being hospitalized with diabetes than were those who lived near the river but far from a waste site.

But wait. Many of these "persistent organic pollutants" include everyday chemicals present in every home in America, not just the notorious toxins found moldering in toxic dumps or spewing from factories. These days, all it takes to be exposed to persistent organic pollutants, or POPs, is to be alive.

THEY'RE EVERYWHERE

"I guarantee you have some of these chemicals in your body."

David Carpenter, MD, director of the Institute for Health and the Environment at the University of Albany, has authored dozens of studies of environmental risks over the years, including the studies of the Mohawks' Akwesasne reservation and the New York hazardous waste sites.

"If you drink milk that is not skim, if you eat eggs or butter or meat or chicken or fish, you're going to get some of these POP compounds, because they are in fat and they're widely distributed," he told me. "Their manufacture started in the late 1920s, early '30s, and then after World War II they skyrocketed. They were very useful products manufactured in the United States until 1977, when the Environmental Protection Agency outlawed them. The problem is they are very hard to destroy, both in the environment and in the human body. They're a residue of a previous age."

POPs include not only infamous compounds like dioxin, DDT, and PCB, but more exotic ones with names like aldrin, chlordane, dieldrin, endrin, mirex, heptachlor, hexachlorobenzene, toxaphene, tributyltin—and the list just keeps on going. Some were used as solvents, others in pesticides, pharmaceuticals, and paints or in manufacturing processes.

While POP levels have been slowly sliding, both in the environment and in people, one of their peculiar and unfortunate tendencies is to accumulate in fat, so that their levels rise with the food chain, particularly in seafood, as little fish get eaten by bigger fish—and most strongly in fatty fish like salmon and tuna. When Carpenter studied how often a person could safely eat salmon while staying within EPA recommendations for dioxin, PCBs, and other contaminants, he concluded that farmed salmon from North America could be eaten at most once per month, while farmed salmon from northern Europe had even higher PCB levels, such that only a single serving every five months can be safely consumed. The safe upper limit for wild Pacific salmon, on the other hand, was about once a week.

"I got in trouble with the salmon farming industry for that study," Carpenter said. "The POP levels in those salmon are sky high. But no matter what you eat, it's impossible to avoid some exposure."

What has struck him about the effect of POPs on the risk of diabetes, he said, is how surprisingly strong the association appears to be, for reasons that remain to be elucidated. In the Native Americans he studied, he separated the subjects into three groups, based on the level of PCBs in their blood. "We found that people in the highest third of PCB exposure had a 3.9-fold increased chance of diabetes compared to people in the lowest third of PCB," he said. "Other groups have found even higher risks. We still have a lot to learn, but it's very likely in my estimation that exposure to these compounds has contributed to the increased incidence of diabetes."

In 2003, researchers from Brussels, Belgium, examined the risk of diabetes in 257 people. When they divided them into ten groups based on their levels of various POPs, those with the highest measure of dioxin had just over five times the risk of diabetes as those with the lowest level. Compared to those with the lowest levels of PCBs, the risk of diabetes in those with the highest levels of PCBs was more than 13-fold.

That's far from the highest risk for diabetes seen in a study of POPs, however. That distinction belongs to a study published in 2006 in the journal *Diabetes Care.* It involved a cross-section of 2,016 adults from across the United States who participated in the National Health and Nutrition Examination Survey (NHANES) between 1999 and 2002. Levels of six POPs, including dioxin and DDT, had been measured in the blood of the participants, who had also been asked whether they'd ever been told by a doctor that they had diabetes. After statistically controlling for age, sex, race, poverty, BMI, and waist circumference, the researchers placed the participants into five categories based on their POP levels. Those in the next-to-lowest level of POPs had 14 times the risk of diabetes as those in the very lowest level. Those in the next highest level also had about 14 times the risk. Where things went crazy was in the highest categories of POP exposure. In the fifth and highest level, the risk of diabetes was an incredible *37.7 times higher* than in people with the lowest levels of POPs.

That's not a 37 percent increased risk. It's not even a 370 percent increased risk. *It's a 3,750 percent increased risk.*

Epidemiological studies almost never show risk levels like that. A doubling of risk is considered robust; a fivefold increased risk raises eyebrows. But a 38-fold increase? That's comparable to the effect of cigarette smoking on the risk of lung cancer. That's the kind of thing that catches people's attention.

"I could barely sleep when I learned this," said Duk-Hee Lee, MD, PhD, the South Korean researcher who co-authored the study. "The more important thing was that obesity was not associated with diabetes among persons with very low levels of POPs. In fact, diabetes itself was extremely rare among these persons even though they were very obese."

The article soon generated not one, but two editorials in the prominent British medical journal *The Lancet*. The first, published one month after the publication of Lee's paper, in August of 2006, took particular interest in the study's finding that obesity leads to diabetes *only* when a person has POPs above a certain level. If confirmed, the editorial stated, the finding "might imply that virtually all the risk of diabetes conferred by obesity is attributable to persistent organic pollutants, and that obesity is only a vehicle for such chemicals. This possibility is shocking." In other words, if Lee's findings hold up, the editorial was implying, *it's not the fat that causes type 2, but the POPs in the fat.* That might help to explain why, beyond simple genetic predisposition, so many people who are seriously overweight never develop type 2, and why so many who are only mildly overweight do.

The second editorial, published a year and a half later, in January of 2008, acknowledged that Lee's findings were "a surprise for many people working in diabetes research, because most studies to date have focused on the effects of genetics and the Westernisation of dietary habits and lifestyle, while ignoring the potential effect of" pollutants.

No scientist was more surprised by the findings than Lee herself, who until she decided to undertake the study had never heard of POPs. In fact, she had no particular interest in pollutants; they were outside her specialty. And to this day, she says, "I am sure that most diabetes researchers have never heard of POPs during their lives, like me three years ago."

BUILDING THE HYPOTHESIS

As an associate professor of preventive medicine at Kyungpook National University in Daegu, South Korea, Lee had built herself a nice reputation studying a somewhat obscure molecule with the ungainly name of gamma-glutamyltransferase, or GGT. Best known as a marker of liver dysfunction or alcohol consumption, GGT turns out to be a ubiquitous presence on the outside of nearly all cells in the body, where it recycles a cellular antioxidant called glutathione. Levels of it in the blood appeared to be a marker of oxidative stress. Collaborating with David R. Jacobs, PhD, a professor of public health at the University of Minnesota (they met via email, through a Korean student at his university), Lee showed that as levels of GGT rise, so rises the risk of diabetes. In fact, a study they did involving 4,088 Koreans found that those with the highest levels of GGT in their blood had 25 times greater risk of diabetes than those with the lowest levels. Clearly, this was a remarkably strong predictor.

Some researchers believed that GGT itself was the bad boy causing the oxidative stress and resulting health problems directly, but Lee suspected that it was merely a bystander, a marker, of something else bad going on. Adding to the mystery was another study by Lee and Jacobs, involving 8,072 Korean men, showing that the average GGT level had more than doubled between 1996 and 2003. What could be driving this increase in GGT numbers? Lee guessed that perhaps the culprit was some kind of environmental toxin. But which?

"There are lots of pollutants," Lee told me by email. "What kinds of pollutants can explain the association between serum GGT and diabetes? I thought that this pollutant should satisfy several conditions." First, it had to be widespread, probably something eaten. Second, it had to be fat soluble, because GGT levels go up with obesity. And third, it had to be something that could be metabolized with the assistance of GGT, since why else would GGT levels go up in its presence? "After reviewing a broad range of books and articles, I finally came to know about POPs," she told me. POPs, she realized, satisfied all three conditions, because they are carried in food; they are stored in fat; some require GGTs to be metabolized; and prior studies had shown that as people were exposed to them, GGT levels went up.

"Even though I hypothesized that POPs may explain the association between serum GGT and type 2 diabetes," she told me, "I soon realized that testing this hypothesis by myself would be difficult because the measurement of POPs is very expensive and requires large amounts of serum. I did not have a research fund for studying POPs."

After months of disappointment, Lee learned that NHANES included laboratory measures of POPs. Within a week of getting their hands on the NHANES data and finding the extraordinary 38-fold increased risk of diabetes in those with the highest levels of POPs, Lee and Jacobs had written their groundbreaking paper that would appear in *Diabetes Care*. Since then, they have also shown that increased levels of POPs are associated with heart disease, periodontal disease, and in women, rheumatoid arthritis. The last is of note because rheumatoid arthritis is, like type 1 diabetes, an immune disorder.

"I have suspected that type 1 diabetes is also related to POPs, because POPs appeared to disturb our immune system," Lee told me. "Even though there is no concrete evidence on type 1 diabetes yet, it would be highly plausible."

She and Jacobs have been steadily building their case for the POP hypothesis, publishing papers in such leading journals as *Diabetes* and *Diabetologia*. Still, some in the field remain skeptical.

"I don't have any disagreement with there being an association there," said Matthew P. Longnecker, MD, ScD, head of the Biomarker-based Epidemiology Group at the National Institute of Environmental Health Sciences, when I reached him at his office in Research Triangle Park, North Carolina. "But when you ask how strong the evidence is for a causal relation, that's where I feel like it's not so clear."

Although Longnecker published three papers about the possible relationship between POPs and diabetes long before Lee and Jacobs's papers were published, he sees little progress being made on fundamental scientific questions. For one, why would extremely high exposures to POPs—such as during the industrial accidents that led to contaminations in Seveso, Italy, and with the Yucheng survivors in Taiwan—result in only modestly increased rates of diabetes, and *only in women,* whereas more routine exposures in the United States, as seen by Lee and Jacobs, result in extraordinarily high rates for *both sexes?*

"These people in Taiwan got an absolutely whopping dose of PCBs," Longnecker told me. "They were poisoned with it. But the men didn't get more diabetes, and the women had just a twofold increase. It doesn't make any sense that a huge dose causes this modestly increased risk only in women, and then you're talking about infinitesimal doses in the NHANES data with a 38-fold increased risk. There's something really odd."

It could be argued that Lee and Jacobs's analysis of the NHANES data is in fact a more accurate measure of the effect of POPs than those in prior studies, because they were the first to make use of actual blood levels of POPs rather than just presumptions of exposure based on geographical exposures. But Longnecker raises a more fundamental question, for which there is as yet no good answer: What if people prone to diabetes simply tend to soak up POPs more readily than others, or are less efficient at excreting them? The buildup of POPs in their bodies might then actually be an *effect* of diabetes, rather than a *cause.*

"People with diabetes may metabolize these compounds differently," he said. "I'd say a healthy measure of skepticism is well founded."

CAUTION CHILDREN

For his part, Jacobs agrees that much remains to be proved. When he and Lee first found that contaminants could increase the risk of diabetes 38-fold, he told me, "I guess I thought that was extraordinary.

We don't see very many things like that in epidemiology. I thought it might be an overstatement. Taken literally, it would be truly revolutionary. But it should be taken with a grain of salt. Do I think POPs cause diabetes? I think they might. But I'm not willing to say we have the evidence yet to prove that they absolutely do."

Greater certainty should come from a study he and Lee are now working on in collaboration with the CDC. They're analyzing blood samples taken from people back in the mid-1980s to check for POP levels, then following up to see who among them developed diabetes over the following two decades. Such before-and-after studies, with the exposure preceding the diabetes by years, could help close the case for causality.

While awaiting the results, I asked Lee what if anything people can do to limit their exposure to these contaminants.

"POPs are bioaccumulated in the food chain," she told me. "Thus, I think that animal foods may be more harmful than plant foods. The fatty part of animal foods would be more harmful. However, even plant foods can be contaminated with POPs. Importantly, even though organochlorine pesticides were banned in developed countries several decades ago, some of them are still used in developing countries in Asia, Africa, or maybe Latin America. DDT [a powerful pesticide that was banned in the United States in 1972] is still used for control of malaria. So, imported food can be harmful. Consumption of locally grown and organic foods may be important."

Not all contaminants, of course, persist for years in the human body like POPs do. The chemical bisphenol-A, or BPA, is widely used to make plastics harder and to prevent rusting and bacteria within food and beverage cans. Because it mixes easily with water (unlike POPs, which prefer fat), most of the tiny amount of BPA that enters the body is quickly excreted in the urine. Yet in 2008, researchers from Britain and Iowa reported in the *Journal of the American Medical Association* that people with high levels of BPA—as seen, once again, in the NHANES database—had a 39 percent increased risk of diabetes, and a similarly increased risk of heart disease.

The study drew a flood of news coverage, not to mention serious push-back from the chemical industry, which pointed out that no clear proof that BPA actually *causes* the diseases had been established. But with other studies linking BPA to cancer and neurological damage, lawmakers in Minnesota, Connecticut, and Chicago took action in May of 2009 to outlaw the chemical in certain food containers. The following month, the FDA announced it would reconsider whether levels of BPA currently found in hard plastic bottles are safe.

And what of TCE and PCE, the contaminants in Woburn that caused leukemia in dozens of people? Their half-lives are only a few days, Lee told me, but unlike BPA, they are fat soluble, which means they might build up in people's fat tissue. "I think that TCE and PCE may be also regarded as kinds of POPs," she said. "These compounds are certainly organic, man-made (hence pollutants), and have some perhaps weak properties of persistence."

Unless and until more research is conducted, Kris and Greg Ahearn and other residents of Woburn will remain uncertain whether the "cancer water" that flowed in the town's wells prior to the 1980s had anything to do with the cluster of cases of type 1 diabetes.

After meeting with Kris and Greg, I drove over to the Goodyear School, where their sons had been students when they were diagnosed. The original 82-year-old building, a square brick cracker box, had been added onto in stages and phases with no apparent signs of a plan—a wing here, a retrofitted trailer there. Named after Charles Goodyear, who lived in Woburn as he was perfecting the process of vulcanizing rubber, the school was slated for demolition and in its final year of use. Plans were underway for a new school to be built in a nearby park, until tests found traces of arsenic in the groundwater there. Arsenic, a potent poison, has also been linked to an increased risk of type 2 diabetes at trace levels.

Before leaving town, I decided to take a look at the old neighborhood where Kris grew up, and where Cheryl Beasley and Tammie Brinkley still live with their children. Located just uphill from the

Aberjona River, once liberally used by dozens of tanneries and other businesses to carry off their waste, the neighborhood nevertheless retains some old-fashioned American charm. The streets are small, with plenty of big, beautiful trees forming a leafy canopy overhead. The modest homes are built close together, some lovingly cared for, others not so much. A big-screen TV can be seen glowing in the living room of one home; another has an old refrigerator and washer sitting beside it. And planted beside the curb, three of them in the span of two short blocks, are rectangular yellow street signs, now dented and rusted, each showing the black silhouette of a child running between a simple two-word warning: "Caution Children."

CHAPTER 8

The Sunshine Hypothesis

How Too Little Sun, and Too Little Vitamin D, Might Raise Diabetes Risk

N EXT ON THE LIST of possible culprits in the rising rate of diabetes is something that Weston, Woburn, other suburbs of Boston, and the rest of the northern United States (not to mention all of northern Europe, Asia, and Russia) have way too little of during the winter: sunshine of sufficient intensity to generate the natural production of vitamin D in the skin. More than three decades ago, before our era of paranoia over the risks of getting too much sun, two brothers discovered the risk of getting too little.

It was June of 1974 when the brothers, Cedric and Frank Garland, took a cross-country road trip from their home in San Diego to Baltimore. They drove a 1970 white Mustang with red-and-blue striping. Frank had just turned 24, Cedric was not yet 28, and they both were single.

"It was a hot-looking car," Cedric told me recently. "Very powerful. We had a great time with it."

As they neared the city of New Orleans, what captured their imagination was not the prospect of carousing, or picking up girls, but how the quality of sunlight had fallen off, blocked by clouds and pollution, since crossing east of the Mississippi. "It was a dramatic contrast to the bright blue air back in the West," Cedric said. "We commented on it repeatedly. We could see this brown cloud over New Orleans. Every other city after that, the sky over it would be gray or brown or yellow."

Cedric had something of an interest—"I guess you could call it a preoccupation"—with the sun. It had begun when he was ten years old, in 1957, when the International Geophysical Year brought countless news reports about new investigations into sun spots, the aurora, the ionosphere, and other Earth sciences. "Our father was a lover of science," he said. "To him the International Geophysical Year was the biggest thing that ever happened. It just caught his fancy. He accumulated every article on it. My brother and I became just terribly interested in it."

Frank remembers it a tad differently. "Cedric was very interested," he told me. "I was seven years old. My brother is the great brain. He is a true genius and has always been recognized for that. Cedric might read a book about butterflies; I would have been outside catching them."

Indeed, Cedric had enrolled at the University of Southern California at the age of 15, and was heading now, in the summer of 1974, to take a new job as assistant professor of epidemiology at Johns Hopkins University. Frank, who had just received a bachelor's degree from the University of California at Los Angeles, was joining him to attend Johns Hopkins as a postgraduate student in the same department.

Within days of their arrival, the brothers attended a noon seminar together. Robert Hoover, MD, an epidemiologist at the National Cancer Institute, had been invited to give a talk about the distribution of cancer in the United States. It was early in July, stultifyingly hot, and the air conditioner wasn't working in their second-floor classroom.

The Garlands missed San Diego; they hated the weather in Baltimore and wondered why they had ever come out East.

And then, with the blinds lowered and the lights turned off, Dr. Hoover showed a slide of a United States map with county-by-county rates of colon cancer. Each county was shaded on a scale from red to blue, depending on whether its rate was high (red) or low (blue). Looking at the pixilated image, Cedric noticed the same general pattern that was obvious to others: it was redder in the North, particularly the Northeast, and bluer in the South. The reason for such a gradient had led to much speculation among other epidemiologists, but to Cedric it was instantly and stunningly obvious. He leaned over to his brother, looked him straight in the eye, and said, "I think it has something to do with the sun."

Remembering it decades later, Cedric told me, "There's no question that at that single moment, the next thirty-five years of our lives were set in motion. We became collaborators from that day forward to this day."

The brothers embarked on a study that was published six years later, in the September 1980 edition of the *International Journal of Epidemiology*. "It is proposed that vitamin D is a protective factor against colon cancer," they wrote. (Known as the "sunshine" vitamin, vitamin D is synthesized from cholesterol in the skin, in response to sunlight.) "This hypothesis arose from inspection of the geographic distribution of colon cancer deaths in the U.S., which revealed that colon cancer mortality rates were highest in places where populations were exposed to the least amounts of natural light—major cities, and rural areas in high latitudes. The hypothesis is supported by a comparison of colon cancer mortality rates in areas that vary in mean daily solar radiation penetrating the atmosphere."

At first more or less ignored by the cancer establishment, the Garland brothers kept pounding away at the subject. In 1985, Cedric co-authored a study in *The Lancet* using a survey conducted in the late 1950s with 1,954 men who had completed detailed diaries of everything they'd eaten for a month. Nineteen years later, those who'd been in the bottom quartile of vitamin D and calcium consumption had a 3.8 percent risk of being diagnosed with colorectal cancer, compared to 1.4 percent in the top quartile—a difference of nearly two-thirds.

But diary reports of food intake are notoriously unreliable, so the Garlands mounted a study of diabolical exhaustiveness. This time, using blood samples drawn from 25,620 volunteers, they measured the actual serum levels of vitamin D. People with the lowest levels of vitamin D in their blood, the brothers found, had *five times the risk of developing colon cancer* as those with the highest levels, according to the study they published, again in *The Lancet,* in 1989.

"That was a pretty definitive study in a worldwide journal," Cedric reflected. "It was the first time anyone had ever collected twenty-five thousand samples of blood to store away for a study."

The brothers continued their studies, soon finding evidence of the same remarkably strong benefit of sun exposure and vitamin D levels on cancers of the breast and ovaries. They figured the American Cancer Society would begin a major campaign to get the word out on the importance of taking vitamin D supplements, but to this day the ACS makes no recommendation. As Dr. Marji McCullough, strategic director of nutritional epidemiology at the ACS, told me, "The Garlands' ecological studies and those of others have sparked a lot of interest. Right now we're awaiting the results of randomized trials. Whether we would specifically recommend vitamin D for cancer prevention, I think the jury is still out."

The Garlands and others have since linked increased sun exposure, vitamin D levels, or both to dramatic reductions in the risk of cardiovascular disease, multiple sclerosis, Alzheimer's disease, Parkinson's disease, and schizophrenia. And then someone asked Frank to give a lecture about a topic he knew little about: the epidemiology of diabetes.

SHEDDING LIGHT ON DIABETES

As Frank investigated the question of vitamin D and diabetes, he came upon a startling study from Finland. In 1966, all 12,055 women who gave birth in Oulu and Lapland, in northern Finland, participated in a survey. Because the country receives so little sunlight compared to more southern nations, Finland at the time recommended that parents give their children a relatively high daily dose of vitamin D—2,000 IU (a standard measurement of vitamins)—in order to prevent the bone-softening disease rickets. The survey, carried out over the first year of the newborn babies' lives, asked mothers how often they gave the recommended vitamin D supplement—daily, occasionally, or never—and how much they gave.

Thirty years later, a young Danish researcher named Elina Hyppönen, PhD, asked the children, by then grown, for permission to do a follow-up survey matching their vitamin D intake to their risk of ever getting type 1 diabetes. Compared to their non-diabetic peers, Hyppönen found, those with diabetes were over eight times more likely to have never received vitamin D. Even among those who were given the supplement regularly, the ones who received the recommended dose of 2,000 IU had about one-fifth the risk of developing type 1 as did those who received less. That is, a simple daily vitamin pill had cut children's risk of diabetes by nearly 80 percent.

Hyppönen's study, published in November 2001 in *The Lancet,* was hardly the first to show a link between vitamin D intake and the risk of type 1 diabetes, but hers made the link impossible to ignore by serious academics. Researchers had already shown by then that type 1 could be prevented in mice by giving them vitamin D_3, and other European studies had seen a similar effect.

"Vitamin D is a very attractive hypothesis," said Arlan Rosenbloom, MD, a nationally recognized type 1 researcher at the University of Florida College of Medicine in Gainesville. "It's consistent with some good epidemiologic data."

Hans Åkerblom, the Finnish doctor who has long pursued the cow's milk hypothesis, agreed that the evidence for vitamin D having an effect on the risk of type 1 is compelling. "Of course vitamin D and sun exposure should be studied," he told me. "It's very likely that type 1 diabetes is not due to one single factor, but a combination of several. Cow's milk could be one of them. Height and weight as risk factors are also interesting phenomena."

Indeed, studies have shown that vitamin D might also prevent or improve the treatment of type 2. Decreased circulating levels of vitamin D have been linked to decreased insulin *secretion* and increased insulin *resistance;* British researchers even found that people with low levels of vitamin D had high blood-sugar levels ten years later. Perhaps the most powerful study of type 2 and vitamin D, however, came in 2006, in the journal *Diabetes Care.* Using data from the Nurses Health Study, involving 83,779 women followed for 20 years, researchers from Tufts and Harvard compared those who took at least 1,200 milligrams of calcium and 800 IU of vitamin D each day to those who took less than half that dose. After controlling for potentially confounding variables (such as income and other health conditions), they found that women who took the higher doses had a 33 percent lower risk of developing type 2 compared with those who took less calcium and vitamin D.

Think about it: there is no known toxicity from vitamin D at 800 IU. Indeed, as noted above, there is no known toxicity at 2,000 IU. And there is no drug now on the market that has ever been shown to reduce the risk of developing type 2 diabetes over a 20-year period, let alone reduce the risk of type 1.

Despite the research findings, however, no increase in recommended vitamin D intake has come so far from government agencies. Today, neither Finland nor the United States—nor any other country—recommends the daily 2,000 IU for infants or children that the Hyppönen study found to have such a powerful preventive effect. In

1975, in fact, Finland *cut* its recommended daily allowance to 1,000 IU, and cut it again, to 400 IU, in 1992. During that same period, Finland's annual incidence of newly diagnosed cases of type 1 soared, from about 15 of every 100,000 children under the age of 14 in the early 1960s to more than 65 per 100,000 today—the highest recorded rate in the world.

In the United States, the minimum recommended daily intake of vitamin D is only 200 IU from birth to age 50, a level chosen primarily to avoid bone diseases. Yet since the findings on vitamin D and other diseases have emerged, the average level of vitamin D in the blood, as measured in an ongoing U.S. study, has actually fallen—from 30 nanograms per milliliter in the late 1980s and early 1990s to 24 ng/mL a decade later. "These findings have important implications for health disparities and public health," the authors of the study wrote in the March 2009 edition of the *Archives of Internal Medicine*. "This drop was associated with an overall increase in vitamin D insufficiency to nearly three of every four adolescent and adult Americans." Five months later, another study, published in the journal *Pediatrics,* found that an astonishing seven out of ten children in the United States now suffers from a vitamin D insufficiency.

What could explain such a sudden drop in vitamin D levels? Yet another recent study, published in the *Proceedings of the National Academy of Sciences,* suggested a possible answer: *videophilia,* defined as "a preference for indoor media activities over outdoor recreation." Since 1991, during the rise of video games and the Internet, per-capita visits to U.S. parks dropped between 18 percent and 25 percent, the study found. "There's a real and fundamental shift away from nature—certainly here [in the United States] and possibly in other countries," said one of the study's authors, Oliver Pergams, visiting research assistant professor of biological sciences at the University of Illinois at Chicago. "The replacement of vigorous outdoor activities by sedentary, indoor videophilia has far-reaching consequences for physical and mental health, especially in children."

Even for those who do venture outdoors, the amount of vitamin D synthesized by their skin will depend on the distance they live from the equator. And, as it happens, their global positioning has a systemic effect on the risk of developing type 1 diabetes, according to a 2007 study in *Diabetologia*. In sunny spots like Cuba, Peru, and Bermuda, the annual incidence of type 1 is under five per 100,000 children. Chillier climes tend to have far higher rates. On the southernmost tip of South America, for instance, Tierra del Fuego's rate is about 20 per 100,000; at the other tip of the globe, Sweden's rate is close to 30 per 100,000. The association is not perfect, with sun-soaked Sardinia having a rate nearly as high as Finland's, and the frosty Netherlands having a rate lower than Kuwait's. But overall, among 52 countries included in the study, distance from the equator is strongly associated with risk of diabetes.

But who ever would have thought to carry out a study mapping diabetes against sun exposure?

GARLANDS GARNER NO GARLANDS

"In Boston, you cannot make any vitamin D from November through March, even if you were standing naked in the middle of the city."

So Frank Garland, PhD, once told a reporter for the *New York Times*, years before his and Cedric's global diabetes study was published. Now director of science planning at the Naval Health Research Center, the Department of Defense's leading epidemiologic research institution, Frank remains as shocked by the diabetes establishment's failure to get the word out about the value of vitamin D as he was, 30 years ago, by the cancer establishment's lack of action. Just talking about Dr. Elina Hyppönen's study in Finland, and the fact that no change in government recommendations for vitamin D followed from it, gets the pitch of his voice rising.

"What did they do the study for if they're just going to recommend that people continue taking forty IU?" he said. "At least go up to the level where no adverse effects have ever been seen, to two thousand IU. Do they think these numbers are just blips on a screen, that they mean nothing? This incredible epidemic of diabetes has occurred there, from fifteen per 100,000 to sixty-five, and they're going to say, 'further research is warranted'? That's what shocks me. To me an epidemic like that is a public health crime. It has to be dealt with. That's our job, not to dance all around it."

Cedric, now a gray-haired professor of family and preventive medicine at UC–San Diego, shares his younger brother's capacity for seeing the numbers and statistics they discuss for the lives and suffering they represent. "Diabetes could be considered an academic problem," he told me. "That's how it is to some people. 'Gee, that's interesting; diabetes can be prevented with vitamin D.' To me, the sense of urgency is imminent. I would feel my life had not been fulfilled if I weren't able to convince the diabetes community of the importance of this. Did you know even within the United States, there's a sixfold difference in the incidence of type one between northern states, like Minnesota and Wisconsin, and southern places like San Diego and Hawaii? My opinion is that virtually all of type one diabetes is due to a deficiency of vitamin D. When you look at the data, there's no other explanation that fits. This is not a hard disease. It appears to be a single-factor disease, and the factor is the vitamin D deficiency. Once we address it, we'll ask why it took so many centuries."

But wait a minute: wasn't vitamin D supposed to be just for building bones? What makes it so special that it can prevent diabetes and cancer and, like, everything else?

"Vitamin D is a vitamin, but it's really closer to a steroid hormone," Frank told me. "Almost every cell in the body has a receptor for vitamin D, and it's essential to life. That's an amazing thing."

One of its most important roles, they believe, is to act as a kind of cement to maintain tight junctures between the epithelial cells that line the inside of the gut, lungs, and blood vessels and make up much of the endocrine glands—including the pancreas. "When these tight junctions are maintained," Cedric explained, "it prevents viruses or harmful enzymes going between them. We think when vitamin D is low, this barrier function that protects the delicate beta cells from viral attack can be penetrated. Another factor is that vitamin D up-regulates an interesting kind of white blood cell, a tolerogenic lymphocyte."

Could he translate that, please?

"It's a peacemaker in the immune system," he said. "It goes to where there's an autoimmune attack, and will modulate or stop the attack. It probably rescues some children in the summer from developing diabetes, when their vitamin D levels go up."

I asked him whether randomized trials need to be carried out, to prove the benefit of vitamin D beyond question and to establish the optimal doses, before parents and policy-makers should consider it for children at risk of developing type 1 (due to having a first-degree relative).

"I'd love to see those studies done," Cedric said. And, in fact, the National Cancer Institute already has better than a dozen studies of vitamin D's anticancer potential underway. But, he added, "The association between smoking and cancer was never tested in a clinical trial. There are conclusions so self-evident that you would not want to do the trial. A trial of type 1 should be done, but the evidence is so unmistakable that vitamin D affects the risk for it that we shouldn't be waiting for a trial."

One large, randomized trial's results have already been published, although it had nothing to do with type 1, or even diabetes. The Women's Health Initiative involved 36,282 postmenopausal women; it was the same study that famously discovered, to the shock of many, that taking estrogen actually increased the risk of breast cancer. It also randomized half of the women to receive 1,000 milligrams of calcium and 400 IU of vitamin D, and half to take an identical-looking placebo. After seven years, those who had been given the calcium–vitamin D combination had a 9 percent lower risk of death than those who had been given the placebo. But the effect was so modest as to be statistically insignificant, even though it was in the right direction. To Cedric and Frank, however, the dose was so small as to have doomed the study from the outset.

What, in their opinion, would be the proper dose to prevent diabetes and other diseases? "The National Academy of Sciences set the safe upper limit at one thousand IU per day for infants up to twelve months, and two thousand IU for anyone older," Cedric told me. "It has no known adverse health effects. I take two thousand IU myself. That's the upper limit. I don't see a good reason for me to exceed it, or to take less." He emphasized that vitamin D_3 is the preferable form, since D_2 is far less potent. And, he added, "Men should also consume one thousand milligrams of calcium, and women should take twelve hundred of calcium. Vitamin D needs calcium to produce its full effectiveness, whether for rickets or cancer, and I'm pretty sure it will be true for diabetes."

Prescribing sun exposure is a trickier proposition, given the risks of skin cancer. "I get five to ten minutes of sunlight very day when the weather allows," Cedric said. "It's not easy. The days that I do, I take a walk during lunchtime. If I can get far enough away from the office, I'll just have an undershirt on. If I had my choice, I would say workers should be provided leisure places where they can get in a swimming pool or get out into the sun."

FEARING THE LIGHT

I have two excellent, personal reasons for violently rejecting the sunshine hypothesis. First, I am a survivor of the most lethal type of skin cancer, melanoma. Second, my previous book, *Natural Causes*, was about the lack of proven benefits, and evidence of multiple health risks, associated with all kinds of dietary supplements and vitamins. With that kind of résumé, you would think I'd be the last person to consider sunshine or vitamin D as a means of preventing anything.

So indulge me this moment of self-congratulation for having written, on page 180 of the hardcover edition of *Natural Causes,* the following (and I quote):

> Almost drowned out amid the white noise of unsubstantiated claims comes, sotto voce, the case for vitamin D, which just may be the only vitamin that the average American needs *more* of. In February of 2005, the *Journal of the National Cancer Institute* published two studies showing that increased exposure to sunlight is linked to increased survival in melanoma patients, as well as a lowered risk of developing lymphoma. According to an editorial accompanying the studies, the effect was likely due to vitamin D, which the skin makes in response to sunlight.

Actually, in that book as in this, I simply did my best to follow the evidence and tell what I learned. Vitamin D looked good then; it looks good now. And as for my own case of melanoma (which was quite tiny, thin, and in the earliest, least dangerous stage), I certainly am a poster boy for the usual risk factors: I had some severe sunburns during summers at the Jersey shore when I was growing up in the 1960s; I am fair and freckle-faced; and my work as a writer has kept me mostly indoors except on weekends and holidays.

I was shocked to learn from the Garlands, however, that the kind of routine, brief sun exposure they have found to prevent other cancers also appears to prevent melanoma, and to increase the chances of survival if a person does get it.

"We did a study of Navy personnel in 1990," Cedric told me. "We thought the construction workers would be the ones who'd have all the melanoma, and the sonar operators, who are inside all day, would be at the lowest risk. We found the indoor workers had the same risk as the outdoor workers. But those in the middle had the lowest. If you had no sun or a huge excess, you had more risk. But not if it was a more balanced exposure."

More recently, a 2005 study in the *Journal of the National Cancer Institute* found that a history of sunburn and high intermittent sun exposure actually increased the chances that a person diagnosed with melanoma would survive it. More recently, a 2008 study in the *European Journal of Cancer* found that people who had routinely spent time at the beach prior to receiving a diagnosis of melanoma had significantly improved chances of surviving it.

The Garlands are internationally recognized for making the case that the use of sunscreens may actually increase the risk of skin cancer, because while they all protect against UVB radiation, many do not protect against UVA, the kind linked to melanoma. They encourage people to limit their sun exposure to the amount that produces no reddening: about five or ten minutes per day for most people, depending on skin type.

Beyond that, they say, it's best to cover up with either a tightly woven fabric or the proven UVA blocker titanium dioxide. At the same time, however, they're adamant about recommending small daily doses of sun, in addition to vitamin D supplements, as a means for preventing diabetes and other diseases.

"The sun does contain potential for harm," Cedric said. "If you get a squamous or basal cell carcinoma on your nose, surgery can be difficult. But if you get it anywhere else on your body, surgery is very easy. So protect your face. Take your shirt off if your circumstances allow it. A few minutes per day taking your shirt off would be a good idea. You don't want it to even turn pink. For someone very fair, that might be only three minutes. For someone with a Mediterranean complexion, it might be fifteen minutes. Usually it's no more than ten."

Although their views were considered heretical, even dangerous, back in the early 1980s, today quite a few academics have come around to the Garlands' point of view. At the 2005 American Association for Cancer Research meeting in Anaheim, California, Edward Giovannucci, MD, professor of medicine and nutrition at Harvard, devoted his keynote lecture to the benefits of vitamin D. "I would challenge anyone to find an area or nutrient or any factor that has such consistent anti-cancer benefits as vitamin D," he told the group. "The data are really quite remarkable." The talk even prompted Michael J. Thun, MD, chief epidemiologist at the American Cancer Society, to urge the society to reconsider its guidelines on sun protection.

Although no formal endorsement of vitamin D for preventing type 1 has yet come from either the American Diabetes Association or the Juvenile Diabetes Research Foundation, a consensus appears to be developing. Among researchers studying the subject, by far the most prolific has been Roger A. Bouillon, MD, PhD, professor of experimental medicine at Catholic University in Leuven, the Netherlands. Since 1985, he has published 34 studies on vitamin D and diabetes, most of them involving rats or mice.

He has found that a deficiency of the vitamin early in life more than doubles the likelihood that mice with a genetic propensity toward type 1 will actually develop it, while mice given extra vitamin D had just one-seventh the risk of developing type 1 as those fed a normal diet.

"There are enough data to conclude that vitamin D supplements can protect beta cells," Bouillon wrote in 2002. "We ... urge especially the parents of children with a higher risk for type 1 diabetes (e.g., first-degree relatives) to adhere to these supplements and to avoid even marginal vitamin D deficiency."

The Garlands even believe that vitamin D might have a more targeted role, in slowing or stopping the destruction of the last remaining insulin-producing cells in a newly diagnosed type 1.

"Many children and adults have a honeymoon period immediately after their diagnosis, where they still have beta cells and don't need to take much insulin," Cedric said. "If we could get vitamin D into those children, they might be able to take less insulin for the rest of their lives. It could arrest the disease process before it plays out. We think it's the best hope for rescuing the incipient case of type one in the honeymoon period."

Speaking of honeymoons, neither of the Garland brothers has ever married. They still live together, along with their ailing mother, in a home not two miles from the sun-drenched coast of La Jolla. More than 35 years after they took that cross-country drive to Baltimore, they relentlessly devote themselves to researching the benefits of vitamin D and continue their long wait for the world to see the light.

CHAPTER 9

The Hygiene Hypothesis

The Icky Benefits of Dirt, Germs, and Worms

A SK THE AVERAGE PERSON what might prompt a cluster of children living in the same neighborhood to develop type 1 diabetes at the same time, and you will probably *not* hear anything about weight, cow's milk, pollutants, or vitamin D. Rather, you're likely to hear the same thing many of the folks I interviewed told me, including those in the Boston suburbs where so many cases have recently popped up.

"Maybe the kids caught a virus or something," said Tammie Brinkley of Woburn.

"My theory of why it's clustered," said Linda Smith of nearby East Taunton, whose daughter Shannon has it, "is because of a virus. Maybe it's a certain strain of virus that comes through, and it triggers diabetes in the people who catch it."

"I do wonder if there's some virus out there," said Patricia Hoban, a nurse in the Weston public schools.

The theory that a virus or bacterium causes type 1 diabetes, especially when the disease occurs in clusters, is the golden oldie of the field, the best known and most widely reported. Literally thousands of news articles have been published on the subject, based on many hundreds of studies that have pursued tantalizing clues that one infectious agent or another attacks the pancreas or kick-starts an autoimmune attack, and that the clusters spread as the virus or bacterium jumps from one child to another. The theory strikes many as so plausible as to be positively self-evident. After all, epidemics are caused by infectious agents, aren't they?

The theory first gained traction over four decades ago, in 1968, when John E. Craighead and Mary F. McLane of the University of Vermont published a study in one of the most respected scientific journals in the world, *Science,* showing that they could cause diabetes in mice by injecting them with a variant of a virus that typically infects pigs and a wide variety of other animals, encephalomyocarditis. Even though the virus had not yet been shown to infect humans, they had proved that a virus could damage the pancreas and raise blood-sugar levels.

Then, in 1969, a British group reported that 123 people who had recently developed type 1 had a high level of antibodies to the Coxsackie B4 (a virus more commonly associated with inflammations of the eye, heart, lungs, and other organs). As additional studies began piling up linking diabetes to Coxsackie, *The Lancet* published an editorial in 1971 predicting the possibility of using a vaccine to prevent diabetes. "British Journal Says Tests Hint Diabetes May Be Caused by One or More Viruses," ran a headline in the *New York Times.* The article quoted researchers calling the findings "fascinating" and "intriguing."

So began a cavalcade of contradictory and inconclusive findings that continues to this day, with as many as 13 other viruses linked to outbreaks of type 1. In 1979, Dr. Ji-Won Yoon and colleagues at the National Institutes of Health reported in the *New England Journal of Medicine* that they had isolated a variant of the Coxsackie B4 virus in the blood of a previously healthy ten-year-old boy three days after he had been hospitalized for diabetes. When they injected mice with the virus, they, too, developed diabetes. An editorial accompanying the study called the findings "highly important." But there was just one catch. Close to *half* of the U.S. population had been exposed at some time in their lives to Coxsackie B4, yet fewer than one in 1,000 at that time had type 1 diabetes. With a "cause" like this, you could say that wearing brown shoes causes diabetes.

Still, scientists and the public fell hard for viruses as the cause of diabetes, and the studies piled up. A study in Erie County, New York, between 1947 and 1967 found that the numbers of new diabetes cases rose and fell with outbreaks of mumps; Allegheny County, Pennsylvania, had a cluster of type 1 cases between 1985 and 1989 following a chicken pox epidemic; Birmingham, Alabama, had one linked to Coxsackie B5 in 1983; and Philadelphia's 1993 uptick in diabetes cases was linked to a mini epidemic, two years earlier, of measles.

But no clear trend ever emerged, and most researchers I spoke to have reached the conclusion that infections are probably little more than the final push over the ledge that results in a case of full-blown diabetes that was already inevitable. Psychological stress, an automobile accent, or any other kind of physical challenge might just as well be the straw that breaks the camel's back. As Johnny Ludvigsson, the Swedish diabetes expert, told me, "Any infection will cause an increased demand for insulin, and I am still convinced that now and then, a virus might directly attack the beta cells. But it has been very disappointing with all these efforts to find 'the' virus that would cause diabetes, like with polio."

But where is it written that every epidemic must be caused by an infection by a microorganism, anyway? Before it became so widely accepted as to seem self-evident, the germ theory was just a theory, one that met with fierce opposition. In 1676, when Antonie van Leeuwenhoek sent the world's first account of single-celled organisms (which he called *animalcules,* or "little animals") to the English Royal Society, they found it so dubious that they sent a team of lawyers and doctors to the Netherlands to look through his microscope for themselves. Well into the 19th century, many scientists continued to believe that infectious agents popped into being out of nothing, a process called spontaneous generation. The germ theory wasn't proved beyond doubt until Louis Pasteur showed that nothing grows in a sterilized flask of broth, so long as it's protected from contamination. Victory against infectious organisms has since vanquished dozens of diseases, extended the human lifespan, and contributed greatly to the extraordinary increase in the human population on Earth.

But what if we have gone too far and been too successful? What if certain infectious agents carry unexpected *benefits* to their human hosts? What if, in the process of seeking protection from van Leeuwenhoek's animalcules, we have created a Dead Zone, leaving our bodies, honed by millennia of unrelenting infectious wars, unprepared for peace? What if the actual *absence* of an infectious agent can cause disease?

What if diabetes can be literally caused by nothing?

HYGIENE BECOMES A DIRTY WORD

In 1963, neurologist David C. Poskanzer and colleagues at Harvard first proposed in *The Lancet* that both multiple sclerosis and polio might be linked to a high level of hygiene. Uri Leibowitz and colleagues at Hadassah University in Jerusalem confirmed this suspicion in a ground-breaking study published in 1966, showing that the risk of developing M.S. was significantly increased among Israelis whose childhood homes had piped water, flush toilets, and fewer than two people per room.

It was not until 1989, however, that the hygiene hypothesis gained a wide scientific following, with the publication of an unassuming, 613-word paper published in the *British Medical Journal* by an epidemiologist named David P. Strachan. The young researcher, then at the London School of Hygiene and Tropical Medicine, had decided to tuck into an old database, called the National Child Development Study, which had been following a group of 17,414 British children born during a single week in March 1958. With no preconceived notion of what he might find, Strachan cross-tabulated 16 different social, environmental, and birth factors to look for any association with their risk of developing hay fever or eczema. Most proved to be dead ends, but one jumped out: firstborn children had a 20.4 percent risk of developing hay fever later in life, while second-borns had a 15 percent risk, third-borns a 12.5 percent risk, fourth-borns 10.6 percent, and fifth-borns 8.6 percent. Likewise, firstborns had a 6.1 percent risk of eczema in their first year of life, compared to just 2.8 percent in fifth-borns.

Why on earth would siblings reduce the risk of hay fever and eczema? Strachan made a leap of insight: kids *without* siblings couldn't get infected by them with the common viruses and bacteria of childhood. Noting that hay fever, asthma, and childhood eczema had all been sharply on the rise in Europe and North America since World War II, he proposed that improved hygiene might have boomeranged on Western civilization.

"Over the past century," Strachan wrote, "declining family size, improvements in household amenities, and higher standards of personal cleanliness have reduced the opportunity for cross infection in young families. This may have resulted in more widespread clinical expression of atopic [allergic] disease, emerging earlier in wealthier people, as seems to have occurred for hay fever."

Although Strachan hadn't actually used the phrase "hygiene hypothesis," hundreds of scientific papers that followed did, and credited him with the original insight. Soon hygiene was being linked in epidemiological and laboratory studies to virtually all the autoimmune diseases whose incidence had risen with the 20th century and skyrocketed after World War II: multiple sclerosis, asthma, allergies, eczema, inflammatory bowel disease, and type 1 diabetes.

Catchy, alliterative, and provocative, the hygiene hypothesis quickly gained a grubby foothold in popular culture. Among parents already predisposed to all things natural—pro-organic, anti-vaccination—the idea that dirt, colds, flus, and other childhood infections were good for their kids seemed, well, natural. Hygiene, in certain quarters, became a dirty word.

But for the scientists, the haziness of the hypothesis has proved something of an obstacle. "We have conducted studies which seem to support the hygiene hypothesis for the development of type one diabetes, and studies which don't," said Chris Cardwell, PhD, a medical statistician at Queen's University of Belfast, Ireland. A 2008 study he co-authored in *Diabetologia* found an increased risk of type 1 in children born by cesarean section (presumably because they were not exposed to naturally occurring bacteria in the course of a vaginal birth). Another showed that children born in remote areas are at increased risk, while a third found that firstborn children are at increased risk.

On the other hand, he has also published a study showing that children with few infections in their first year of life have the same risk of developing type 1 as those with many more infections. "Based upon our data," he told me, "I personally have not reached any conclusions about the hygiene hypothesis."

Other researchers, however, have moved beyond the fieldwork of epidemiology into laboratory experiments to figure out precisely which bacteria or viruses, at which points in the life cycle, might actually have an effect on preventing autoimmune disease. And there the results so far have been impressive.

One of the first such studies, published in 1990 by researchers at the University of Alberta in Canada, involved a strain of mice known as NOD, for "non-obese diabetic," because they develop autoimmune diabetes. The investigators injected 13 mice with complete Freund's adjuvant, a preparation containing the dried, inactivated tuberculosis bacterium, and left 38 untreated. By eight months, all 38 of the untreated mice had died of diabetes, whereas all 13 of the treated mice were still alive, with normal sugar levels, after a year.

In 2002, Japanese researchers reported a similarly preventive effect when they inoculated NOD mice with the bacterium that causes leprosy. Italian researchers reported success in preventing diabetes in NOD mice in 2005 after feeding them a compound called VSL#3, a "pro-biotic" containing the bacterium Streptococcus thermophilus (used in making yogurt) and several species of Lactobacillus (used in beer, cheese, and other foods) and Bifidobacteria. French researchers reported the same effect in 2006 with the injection of the bacterial extract OM-85.

Then, in August of 2008, a truly beautiful study was published in the journal *Nature* by an A-team of researchers from Yale, Cornell, the University of Chicago, the University of California at San Francisco, Bristol University in England, Washington University in St. Louis, and the Jackson Laboratory in Bar Harbor, Maine. To understand the study, one must understand something about NOD mice: they don't develop diabetes in a messy environment. Only with clean water and regularly cleaned cages does their diabetes develop. So the team kept the mouse house nice and clean. But they used a special sub-breed of NOD mice lacking the gene for a protein called MyD88 protein, which the immune system uses to recognize microbes. Even though these mice were raised in a standard, clean environment—the kind that would have led to diabetes in typical NOD mice—most of these special mice still did not develop diabetes. To make them develop the disease, the team had to take another, more drastic step: they gave mother mice antibiotics to kill their gut bacteria, delivered their babies by cesarean section to prevent contamination through the vaginal canal, and then raised the babies in utterly pristine conditions to prevent any of the normal gut bacteria from infecting them. Kept hyper-clean, inside and out, these mice developed diabetes.

Their diabetes, in other words, was literally being caused by nothing, a total lack of bacteria. While Taoists and readers of the *Tao Te Ching* might see in these findings vindication for the proposition that non-being is powerful, the leader of the study described their significance in more earthy terms.

"I don't think it's bad to be a little dirty," said Li Wen, MD, PhD, a senior research scientist in immunology at the Yale University School of Medicine. Reached at her office by telephone, she told me, "People in Africa and other developing regions have an incidence of allergy, asthma, and type one diabetes much lower than in the United States. One reason, we suspect, is that they have such a higher incidence of infectious diseases."

She described the conditions in which they had to raise the specially bred mice in order to get them to develop type 1. "If it's like a four-star hotel, eighty percent of them get diabetes. It's actually better than a four-star hotel. Their food is autoclaved. They're housed in rooms with filtered air. It's all sterile. The human handlers have to be sterile as well. But if they live in the equivalent a cheap motel, the incidence will drop to thirty or forty percent."

So who can't stand some friendly bacteria that help to make yogurt, beer, or just a happy tummy? But of course, bacteria aren't the only little friends humans have carried around with them for eons. For instance, there are head lice. In April of 2009, researchers at the University of Nottingham examined the immune systems of some wild wood mice, comparing those who were heavily infested with lice to those who were lightly infested. The immune systems of those with few lice, they found, were far more trigger-happy toward an autoimmune attack than were the wild mice with lice.

"Much like laboratory mice, people in developed countries are currently exposed to a very different profile of infections to that encountered by their ancestors," said senior author Janette Bradley, professor of parasitology. "Analyzing immune responses in wild populations can give crucial insights into how the immune system functions in its natural context."

Nobody is suggesting that head lice could prevent diabetes, or that anyone would ever want to intentionally acquire head lice. Actually, they're suggesting something much more disgusting.

THE WORM STORY

Incredible—and incredibly repulsive—as it might seem, some of the strongest evidence to date for the hygiene hypothesis involves the benefits of ingesting—*on purpose!*—intestinal worms. If you wonder what kind of a mad scientist could make such a bizarre discovery, allow me to introduce you to Joel V. Weinstock, MD, director of gastro-enterology and hepatology at Tufts Medical Center in Boston.

"Now I'm going to give you the worm story," he began when we started talking, and soon he was on a roll, extolling the wonders of intestinal parasites. "There is an inverse relationship between worming and these immune diseases," he continued. "Everybody had worms in their GI tract in the nineteenth century. They were universal. What we successfully did through modern hygiene is we successfully eliminated exposure to intestinal worms. Jewish kids in the 1930s were the first to start getting Crohn's disease. Well-to-do Jewish kids, who wore shoes and followed Jewish kosher laws. In the 1930s, thirty percent of the American population had been exposed to *Trichinella,* wormy pork. By the middle of the twentieth century, most people were no longer getting worms. They still had bacteria in the gut, but not worms. As it turns out, worms are very, very power-ful inducers of immune regulation. The problem is, I suspect, that hygiene has been good for us. It isn't evil to be clean. What was child-hood mortality in the 1800s? President Lincoln's son Willie died of typhus, from contaminated water. People can now expect to live into their eighties much more readily. But in the process of developing good hygiene practices to protect us from the fifty or so organisms that do us harm, we've deprived ourselves of organisms that do us no harm, and actually help us."

Intestinal worms, Weinstock told me, have co-evolved with humans, learning a neat trick along the way essential for their survival: turning down the molecular rheostat on our immune system, so that our white blood cells don't attack them. So reliant have we become on this process that without the worms, our immune systems, like a car engine idling too high, start going after our lungs (producing asthma), intestines (producing bowel disease), nerve linings (producing M.S.), pancreas (producing diabetes), or other organ systems.

"What if I told you that in the 1800s, nobody had hay fever?" Weinstock said. "It was not a medical disease of the 1800s. The pioneers going across the country in covered wagons didn't worry about hay fever.

"You have a fight side of your immune system to protect you," he went on. "But what would happen if the immune system attacked a bug in your liver and didn't know when to shut down? It has to be able to gate its response. That's what the regulatory side of your immune system does. The theory is that as a result of underexposure to worms and other pathogens, the regulatory immune system is not developing properly." While bacteria and viruses help to "educate" the regulatory immune system, he said, intestinal worms "are probably the most powerful stimulators of our regulatory immune system. That's what they evolved to do. That's their trick. That's why deworming the entire population may have had major consequences."

Still, isn't it more than a little ironic to think that helminths, as intestinal worms are scientifically known, could be anything but harmful and horrifying? The very mention of the word is enough to make most people's faces screw up in revulsion. Search for pictures of them on Google Images, and you'll find a photograph of a man pulling a thin, white, foot-long worm out of a hole in his foot. Search on Wikipedia and you'll end up reading about *Onchocera volvulus,* the worm that causes river blindness and can live for 15 years in the human body. Then there is the African eye worm, the Guinea worm, the Medina worm, the hookworm, and *Wuchereria bancrofti,* which, well, worms its way into the lymph nodes and causes elephantiasis. Or you can check out the study in the journal *Burns* entitled "Airway obstruction by Ascaris, roundworm in a burned child." All of which will make you see why the World Health Organization and charitable groups devote so much time and money to eradicating these nasty little buggers in the estimated one-third of humans infected with them.

But forget about all that, because now we're going to talk about a wonderful, fun, beautiful little worm that hurts nobody, can't be seen, doesn't overstay its welcome, and has a cute little tail that wags like a dog's: the amazing pig whipworm, *Trichuris suis*.

"It's a nice, friendly worm as worms go," said David Elliott, MD, PhD, a gastroenterologist and immunologist at the University of Iowa who has collaborated with Weinstock on whipworm studies. "It was the safest worm we could think of. It's short-lived in humans. It lasts a few weeks and then is gone. You don't need to deworm the person."

In 2003, Elliott and Weinstock took the daring step of asking four people with active Crohn's disease and three with ulcerative colitis if they wouldn't mind downing a refreshing glassful of whipworm eggs. They all agreed to begin with a single dose of 2,500 live *Trichuris suis* eggs. The eggs are far too small to see when taken in liquid; they mature into microscopic whipworms and pass out of the body in a few weeks. All seven patients improved with no apparent side effects; on a quality-of-life index used to measure disease severity, six of them actually went into remission. But the benefits dissipated after a few weeks. Elliott and Weinstock then had two of the Crohn's patients, and two of the ulcerative colitis patients, take the eggs every three weeks for at least 28 weeks. Once again, they experienced remarkable relief from their symptoms, with no apparent side effects.

Because this initial study had no comparison group of people exposed to a placebo treatment, Weinstock, Elliott, and colleagues conducted a larger study, involving 54 people with ulcerative colitis. After 12 weeks, 13 of the 30 people given *Trichuris* eggs had a significant improvement (43.3 percent), compared to four of 24 patients who got a placebo (16.7 percent). While not a home run, in the realm of ulcerative colitis it was a big hit, particularly given that most other treatments carry significant side effects.

"As groups have replicated and extended our work," Elliott told me, "it's now become fairly well accepted that the elimination of helminths may indeed explain why we have all these immune illnesses in developed countries. We don't hear 'that's crazy' anymore."

Another study of *Trichuris* eggs has now been undertaken by John

O. Fleming, MD, director of the Multiple Sclerosis Clinic at the University of Wisconsin Medical School in Madison. At the 2009 American Academy of Neurology meeting in Seattle, he reported that after giving *Trichuris* eggs every two weeks for three months to five M.S. patients, he found no ill effects whatsoever. With support from the National M.S. Society, he is now planning a larger, randomized study in which he will use MRI scans to see whether he can show evidence of a benefit in treated patients.

So promising does the *Trichuris* approach look that the University of Iowa, where Elliott is based, decided to take a patent on it. But where could they find a company that would actually want to base its business model on whipworm eggs?

CORPORATE PARASITES

"My first project was to produce living maggots for treating chronic wounds."

Detlev Goj, the 50-year-old founder of the German firm Ovamed GmbH, had reached me by cell phone. "It's a funny and exciting story, actually," he said in a strong German accent, and let loose with a somewhat maniacal, high-pitched cackle. Despite his evident appreciation for the absurdity of what he had gotten himself into, he turned out to be every bit the serious businessman.

Until 1998, Goj told me, he had been working as marketing manager for the wound care division of a Danish firm, Coloplast. When he heard about research into the use of living maggots on deep wounds (they eat away dead scar tissue as it forms), he proposed commercializing them to his bosses.

"They said, 'This gentleman must be nuts.' So I quit my job and started developing maggots for approval in medical treatment." He founded BioMonde, received European Union approval for the treatment, built up the business, and sold it to a larger firm in 2003. Then he started looking for a new medical business to enter. He took interest in inflammatory bowel disease, for which there are few good treatments, and noticed epidemiological data showing that two of the only places in Europe with low rates of the disease were in small pockets of Germany and France. "Both these places were known for a food specialty, a mite cheese—you can see mites crawling in this cheese."

People eat the mites with the cheese? "You eat them, yes," he said, and cackled again. "My next idea was maybe parasites might have an influence on the development of such diseases. I looked on medical databases. I found a tiny little article from Joel Weinstock having a similar idea, that parasites might have a role in IBD. Then I called Joel Weinstock."

He bought plane tickets to Germany for Weinstock, Elliott, and their colleague, Robert W. Summers. They reached an agreement that Goj would have exclusive license for marketing the patented *Trichuris* eggs. Goj's new firm, Ovamed, has now established a commercial production facility where they grow and prepare the eggs being used in the University of Wisconsin study, and which will also supply a large, multi-center clinical trial of colitis in Europe. Another German firm has paid $8 million for exclusive rights to eventually sell the eggs, if approved, in Europe for the treatment of IBD. Meanwhile, curious consumers can order the eggs from a Thailand distributor.

"To be honest, I treated all my five kids with the therapy already," Goj said. "Not that they have a disease, but for prevention. My youngest daughter, she was three years old when I gave her the therapy. She was developing all kinds of infections at the time, runny nose, tears in the eyes. She caught it almost every other week. I gave her a very low dose, slowly escalating the dose, and she never got sick again. I knew before I gave it to my kids that the worst case that could ever happen is that nothing happens. We have a totally harmless parasite. We are not using the worms, we are using the eggs. If you think about it, people don't mind going into supermarkets eating live yogurt cultures. All we are doing is using a living, microscopic organism, bringing it into the body and letting it stimulate the immune system."

But surely asking people to swallow worm eggs has to be harder than convincing them to permit live maggots to be applied to a serious wound? "Oh the maggots are much worse," he said, again with that high-pitched laugh. "Maggots you can clearly see in your wound crawling, and that's ugly."

Studies of using helminths to prevent type 1 diabetes have also been proceeding, but so far not in humans. The first clear proof that infection with a helminth could prevent diabetes in NOD mice came in 1999. Anne Cooke, a professor of pathology at the University of Cambridge, used *Schistosoma mansoni,* a helminth that infects millions of people worldwide. Feeding either the worm or its eggs to NOD mice, she found, significantly reduced their odds of developing autoimmune diabetes. In 2003, she showed that injecting soluble extracts of the worm or its egg had the same effect, and significantly tempered the animals' immune response. In 2007, she found the same effect from two other intestinal worms, *Trichinella spiralis* and *Heligmosomoides polygyrus.* Most recently, in April of 2009, she again prevented diabetes in NOD mice, this time using only soluble antigens to *Schistosoma* eggs.

"Up until now," she told me, "we have been using crude extracts and have recently started to work with defined molecules provided by our collaborators. I think it is important to identify which molecules are able to provide diabetes prevention and identify the way in which they do so before trying to use such approaches to prevent diabetes. After all you would be giving this to young children. Once we have identified components then I think we could proceed to trial it [in humans]. If you go for an ill-defined extract you run the problem with batch-to-batch variation, and efficacy may not be guaranteed. That would be a big problem as it would destroy faith in something that may have great potential."

So eating the live worms or their eggs might not be necessary after all to prevent diabetes? "We do not need a live infection to get protection from diabetes in NOD mice," she explained. "We feel that it would be more reproducible and palatable to have an isolated product."

How anticlimactic.

In the meantime, while further evidence is gathering on the hygiene hypothesis, Weinstock believes that some safe, prudent recommendations can already be made.

"Do I believe that living in a less hygienic environment could be protective? The answer is yes," he told me. "Children raised on a farm, with large animals, are less likely to get these autoimmune diseases. But what aspect of those exposures are protecting these children is not well defined. Sometimes people ask me, 'Should I take my kids to South America and let them play in a ditch?' That is what I would call an indiscriminate exposure. They could pick up one of the bad boys. They may get hepatitis A. I tell parents of children with immunologic diseases, let your children play in the dirt, have a dog and a cat and don't wash it, let them be exposed to things around them. It's okay to go to a farm and play near the manure. Just common exposures may be helpful, and probably won't be hurtful. Nobody gets sick from playing in the dirt."

APPRAISING THE FIVE HYPOTHOTHES

Then again, who knows how the whole worm story will ultimately pan out as a means of preventing type 1? As more than one researcher told me during the year I spent researching this book, diabetes has been prevented in the NOD mouse dozens of times, yet none of those treatments has yet been proved effective in humans. Maybe worms will be the ticket, or maybe not. Maybe vitamin D or sunshine will be the great breakthrough, or maybe not. Maybe hydrolyzed baby formula, or the elimination of persistent organic pollutants, or a modest reduction in weight will prove beneficial in preventing type 1. Maybe a few of them will ultimately be proved partly effective, and so combining them will be the best step. Or maybe they will all be a bust.

We don't yet know. Until we do, it's reasonable to conclude for now that all of us should be sure we're getting our recommended daily allotment of vitamin D, particularly if we have a first-degree relative with type 1 diabetes. For parents with type 1 who have a newborn child, it's worth keeping in mind that exclusive breastfeeding for the first six months is already recommended by health groups (although doing so can result in a vitamin D deficiency in the infant, so talk to your physician about the possibility of adding a supplement). Parents who wish to give supplemental feedings with a formula might also want to consider whether using a highly hydrolyzed formula, available in most food stores and pharmacies, is worth the extra cost.

To get some perspective on all these potential therapies, and all five of these hypotheses for why diabetes is rising, I decided that the best person to ask would be Judith Fradkin, MD, director of the Division of Diabetes, Endocrinology and Metabolic Diseases at the National Institute of Diabetes and Digestive and Kidney Diseases (NIDDK).

"You wouldn't want to take something based on speculation without proof that it's doing some good," she told me. "All sorts of things are correlated with an increased or decreased risk of type one. But it's very hard to separate out from an epidemiologic study what is actually causative. Just think about all these approaches being studied. Are parents going to give the highest dose of vitamin D to their children? Are they going to give them pinworm eggs, and hydrolyzed formula? You can't do all these things until you have a clinical trial to prove it's safe and effective. I wouldn't be surprised if none of the current hypotheses were right."

To get definitive answers, NIDDK is co-sponsoring The Environmental Determinants of Diabetes in the Young (TEDDY) study, which is in the process of screening a third of a million newborns in the United States and Europe in order to ultimately follow 7,800 children at high risk of developing type 1.

"Using the genomic analysis of stool samples," Fradkin told me, "we may find an unsuspected bacteria or virus that promotes or protects against type one. We're also collecting nasal swabs and a sample of their tap water. We're collecting a lot of samples, and then we'll see who develops diabetes and who doesn't. Whatever the trigger is, we want to find it, because we do think it's environmental. The rates are rising. Something has to be behind it. We need to find it. If we find it, that has tremendous implications for prevention."

She asked me to add one note of caution. "Probably a lot of people reading your book will be parents of children with type one," she said. "Parents of children with any disease can feel very guilty. 'What did I do wrong?' If you say they should have used hydrolyzed formula and vitamin D and all these things, they're going to be blaming themselves and that wouldn't be right. You wouldn't want parents who have kids with type one diabetes saying, 'If only I had done something different.'"

As we await scientific confirmation for or against the five hypotheses described in this second section of the book, Fradkin's concerns are well worth bearing in mind. But now it is time to turn our attention to four practical treatment or prevention strategies, each of them radically different, and each far along toward curing, preventing, or dramatically improving the treatment of type 1 or type 2. They're less about pursuing intellectually provocative theories, and more about doing what works. One involves innovative surgery; another, path-breaking biology; and a third, old-fashioned public health campaigns, dusted off from strategies developed 100 years ago to prevent the epidemics of an earlier generation. First, though, is an approach using automated high-tech gadgetry, in the testing of which I myself participated during a recent clinical trial, freeing me of my diabetes for one wonderful night.

PART THREE

THE REMEDIES

CHAPTER 10

The Computer Cure

The Quest for an Artificial Pancreas

I
T IS THE NATURE of holy grails, in medicine as in religion, that they are much to be desired and never to be obtained.

In March of 2002, an article in the Minneapolis *Star Tribune* stated, "In the world of diabetes research, the artificial pancreas has long been regarded as the Holy Grail." It quoted a past president of the American Diabetes Association as quipping that the quest had gone on "forever," and that success was "still around the corner."

In May of 2006, Aaron Kowalksi, PhD, then director of strategic research projects for the Juvenile Diabetes Research Foundation, was quoted in *USA Today* as calling an artificial pancreas "the holy grail of diabetes."

The following year, in September of 2007, Jennifer Aspy, director of product marketing and operations for Roche Diabetes Care, used the same term, "the holy grail with diabetes," to describe the artificial pancreas in the Pittsburgh *Post-Gazette*.

After nearly two decades as a medical reporter, and almost twice that long as a diabetic, I had long given up on anything called a holy grail or "silver bullet" coming to fruition. Yet in March of 2009, I was scheduled to become one of the first humans ever to sip from this holy

181

grail. For one day and night, I was to be hooked up to a device heralded for years as a breakthrough technology that would virtually cure type 1 diabetes: a fully automated, self-regulating, iPod-like artificial pancreas that would continuously sense my blood-sugar level and release just the right amount of insulin at just the right time, to keep me from going either high or low, without the need for any action, or even awareness, on my part. But before I got my chance—scheduled to begin, strangely enough, on Friday the 13th, in March of 2009—I determined to learn the history of this legendary quest, and perhaps to find its King Arthur.

EARLY DAYS

"The way I got into this business was I realized I had none of the skills I needed to be a catcher for the Yankees."

If anyone can be considered one of the fathers of the modern artificial pancreas, it is William V. Tamborlane, MD, the tan, slim, gray-haired chief of pediatrics at the Yale School of Medicine. Sitting out by the pool of a resort, where he was scheduled to speak at yet another medical meeting, he looked and sounded every bit the patrician Wasp. In fact, Tamborlane told me, he is the grandson of Italian immigrants, who changed the "i" at the end of Tamborlani to an "e." His father, who quit high school during the Great Depression, worked for a while sweeping the floor of a denture factory, where he got it into his head that his sons should become dentists.

"My oldest brother is a dentist," Tamborlane said. "I might have become a dentist too, except a high school counselor said, 'Dentist? Why not be a doctor? You don't have to put your hands in people's mouths all day.'"

By the time Tamborlane had been hired by Yale as an assistant professor of pediatrics and director of its Children's Diabetes Program, in 1977, he already had access to a hulking, oven-sized "glucose-controlled insulin infusion system" sold to hospitals under the name Biostator by the Ames Division of Miles Laboratories in Elkhart, Indiana.

"It was the first closed loop," Tamborlane said, meaning that it was the first system to control an insulin pump automatically, based on measurements of blood-sugar levels. Rather than the pump and the sugar measurements working independently, the two were connected in a continuous feedback loop, with rising sugar levels making the pump release more insulin and falling sugar levels making it release less. "It withdrew blood, ran it through a glucose analyzer, and then secreted insulin. But you had to take one hundred cc of blood out of the patient per day. It was a tabletop thing. "

With no known method for measuring glucose levels without the removal of blood, and the only "portable" insulin pump being the size of a military backpack, the prospects for practical day-to-day use by diabetics looked utterly remote until a young inventor by the name of Dean Kamen entered the fray. Later to gain fame as the inventor of the Segway—yes, the vehicle proclaimed to be the future of transportation, which has turned out to be more the scooter of mall security guards—Kamen had his first big hit with the development of the AutoSyringe, a drug-delivery pump that weighed just over a pound. Originally designed for dialysis, the device was being used in Yale's hematology department when Tamborlane first saw it.

"They called it the Blue Brick," Tamborlane recalled. "It was blue plastic, the size of a brick. That was considered miniaturization in those days. Turns out that Dean Kamen's brother, Bart, was a pediatric resident at Yale. That's how the hematologists got connected to using the pumps. I saw kids wearing this pump. I thought, 'You know, maybe I could use this.'"

In 1978, Tamborlane and three colleagues invited the parents of seven children with type 1 to participate in a study using Kamen's pump to replace injections. "When we had these patients on their usual one or two shots a day, if their sugar levels were under two hundred they were lucky," Tamborlane said. (Under 100 is considered normal.) He calculated an hourly basal rate for the period between meals, and then used the device's red button for giving additional boluses before meals. "The first patient, his peak level after breakfast was like 220. Peak after lunch was 180. Peak after dinner was 150. Peak after the bedtime snack was 120. That's where we discovered you needed more insulin for breakfast than other meals. We fiddled with the diet. The third patient, I had this piece of graph paper. I got the glucose numbers from the hospital lab every hour, just plotting them up. This time, the glucose never went over 140. By that night I was like jumping up and down, clapping. I was a young guy back then. That was thirty years ago. I thought we had solved all the problems of diabetes."

On March 15, 1979, Tamborlane and his colleagues published the results of their study in the *New England Journal of Medicine*. "These results demonstrate that plasma glucose can be lowered to normal in ambulatory patients with brittle juvenile diabetes using a portable, subcutaneous insulin infusion system for two to four days," they concluded.

Soon the AutoSyringe was being sold to diabetics as the first commercial insulin pump. Tamborlane was justly proud, although in retrospect, he realizes those first devices were not nearly as practical as he thought they were.

"I was seeing these happy youngsters wearing their pump around, coming into the clinical research center for their annual checks," he told me. "What I didn't know was because of the size of this device—it was pretty big, it was cumbersome, and you actually had to plug it in and recharge it during the night—a lot of these kids, once they left the hospital, they didn't always use the pump. I'm glad I had this vision of these happy youngsters. If I had known the truth, it might have slowed things down a bit."

Soon a number of companies were selling smaller insulin pumps, and work on a continuous glucose monitor also sped along. But by 2002, progress toward the critical last step—connecting the sensor to the pump with a computer that would decide how much insulin to give based on current sugar levels—remained mired in academic limbo. Which is precisely where it might still be, were it not for a newly minted Internet millionaire whose early retirement at the age of 33 was cut short by a very thirsty son.

THE INTERNET MILLIONAIRE

Jeffrey Brewer was on top of the world. For years he had put in hundred-hour weeks as co-founder of two early Internet juggernauts, goto.com (later renamed Overture, a pioneer of keyword-based advertising and pay-for-placement search results) and citysearch.com. When an initial public offering for Overture was planned in 1998, the investment bankers arranging it suggested that they might want to put it off a few months until Jeffrey, the CEO, turned 30.

"We raised about . . . I think it was a couple hundred million on that IPO," Jeffrey told me. "The day it went public, Overture was worth $1.5 billion. It may have been a little more. Between one and two billion."

We sat around the glass dining room table in the brownstone that he and his wife, Deborah, share with their two children, Sean and Katherine, a black Labradoodle, and a Devon Rex cat (so friendly she walked on my computer keyboard when I stopped typing). The first thing I had seen upon entering the unassuming town house on Manhattan's Upper West Side was a Guitar Hero device hooked to the flat-screen television in the living room; Jeffrey admitted that he played it as much as his son. Tall, thin, and intense, with rimless glasses, Jeffrey wore what Deborah called his "uniform": black shoes, khakis, and a white Oxford shirt.

"I don't even know how we got married; he used to work seven days a week, including Christmas," Deborah said. "We would have family time on Saturday mornings. We would go out for breakfast for three hours. That was it. During the week he would come home between nine thirty and ten. He'd say hello, then the phone would ring. He would spend the next two hours walking around outside and talking on the phone."

In late 2001, having handed off control of Overture and with more than enough money to live on for the rest of their lives, the family set off for a year-long trip to Australia, where Deborah grew up. Upon their return to New York in August of 2002, Jeffrey began looking seriously into charitable work involving Third World economic development. Then they noticed that six-year-old Sean was drinking and peeing a lot. At first they suspected he was just guzzling too much Gatorade. But on September 19, 2002, they took him to the doctor, who, based on a single urine test, announced without hesitation, "Your son has type one diabetes."

As Jeffrey recalled it, "They give us these two types of insulin, Regular and Lente. They showed us this crude sliding scale. 'If this is how high he is, this is how much insulin you give.' I had this log book, I'm testing him every few hours, and I'm thinking, this is crying out for automation. Why do I have to do this? A computer should do this, and will do it better. I was frustrated. Why doesn't this exist, with all that we can do and I'd seen done?"

Flinging himself into the subject with the same intensity he had brought to his Internet start-ups, Jeffrey learned about a group called the Diabetes Technology Society and went to its annual meeting less than a month after Sean's diagnosis. Sitting in the audience during one of the panel discussions, he found himself listening to an arcane academic debate about which kind of computer algorithm would be best for controlling the pump. During the question-and-answer session, Jeffrey stood up and began berating the scientists for dithering over details while children's lives were at stake.

"I was reminding them what this was all for at the end of the day," Jeffrey said. "It seemed eminently doable and it was an obligation of these people to push this forward in an aggressive way. 'We have the pieces here, we need to make progress, we need to start commercializing these technologies, because people living with the disease need it.'"

I asked him where he got the nerve to talk that way to scientists who had devoted their careers to the field, after he had spent just a few weeks dealing with his son's diabetes.

"Being the father of a child with a chronic disease, that gave me a certain credibility and also a certain shield," he explained. But, he added, it was something more. "It was a function of my background, working with engineers, building a business. Even after just a few weeks of measuring blood sugar, administering insulin, and trying to keep this system in balance—God this seemed to be just crying out for automation. I couldn't understand why someone hadn't already done it. There weren't any fundamental scientific problems. The academics had created enough of an opportunity for industry to take over, but industry wasn't aggressively taking over."

Following the meeting, Jeffrey began traveling around the country to visit the offices of the leading manufacturers in diabetes technology, as well as the leading academics. Soon he joined the board of the Juvenile Diabetes Research Foundation. In October of 2004, at another meeting of the Diabetes Technology Society, he pulled a repeat performance of his standing-up-and-dressing-down-a-scientist-from-the-audience routine.

"I can remember it vividly," recalled Aaron Kowalski, who had recently joined the JDRF. "It was amazing. I've been to many, many scientific meetings, and I don't know that I've ever seen anything like that happen. Jeffrey got up and lit into this doctor. 'I completely disagree and you don't understand.' The entire audience started clapping. And then my colleague at JDRF introduced me to Jeffrey."

Kowalksi, a big, friendly guy who is himself a type 1 diabetic (and whose brother also has the disease), quickly realized he had found in Jeffrey a simpatico spirit who shared his vision for pushing forward with the artificial pancreas. JDRF, however, had devoted itself since its founding in the early 1970s to finding a biological *cure*, not a technical *fix*. But Jeffrey was not to be dissuaded. Late in 2004, at a JDRF meeting, he issued his fellow board members a challenge: he would make a donation of $1 million if the organization would make a commitment to seeing an artificial pancreas commercialized. In early 2005, an executive committee of the board told him that JDRF might be willing to be convinced if he would do some due diligence, put together a business plan, and get back to them. Kowalski and Jeffrey became the point men. After months of travel and meetings and investigation, they presented their plan in October of 2005 to the board, which voted to approve it, putting Kowalski in charge of the new initiative.

By July of 2008, the extraordinary progress that had been made in just a few years was in evidence at a state-of-the-art meeting jointly sponsored by the FDA, the NIH, and the JDRF. So, too, however, were lingering frustrations with the remaining roadblocks, from regulatory to computational.

A MODEL OF TRUTH

"One thing I'm hearing from this panel, which concerns me, is I think we're being held up by shooting for perfection."

Just before the first coffee break on Monday morning, July 21, Aaron Kowalski was among the 140 or so scientists, mathematicians, regulators, industrial designers, computer programmers, and patient advocates attending the artificial pancreas meeting on the NIH campus during a blistering heat wave in Bethesda, Maryland. "There is debate on algorithms, there is debate on models, but there are incredibly important steps that a number of us are going to have to take to realize the potential of this technology."

"I agree with you totally," said Bill Tamborlane, who was moderating a session on the latest studies. "If we're waiting for the perfect solution, it's a big mistake. We need to move forward with what we can do now."

A young man stood to speak from the back of the auditorium. "I'm not a doctor, I'm a diabetic," he said. "I can make a lot bigger mistakes in my own control than you show in your results. Why can't something that clearly does it so much better not move forward?"

But most of the scientists at the meeting were plainly not striving to do just a little bit better than people do when they're in control of their own diabetes. Rather, they were shooting for the fine control of blood sugars achieved by healthy insulin-producing beta cells in non-diabetics.

Edward Damiano, PhD, a biomedical engineer at Boston University (whose son was diagnosed with type 1 diabetes a few years ago), described using not only insulin, but also glucagon (the hormone that releases glucose stored in the liver) to keep sugar levels from falling too low. His system required two pumps and two lines going into the patient. "We have no hypoglycemia in our pig studies," he told the attendees. "We're also doing human trials. I'm pretty convinced, having lived with diabetes as long as I have, that glucagon is necessary. It's the counter-regulatory hormone. It's very difficult to show that we can even come close to what our pancreas does without some kind of counter-regulatory balance."

Claudio Cobelli, PhD, professor of bioengineering at the University of Padova in Italy, described what he called "in silico" testing—computer simulations—to bypass the need for animal studies.

Boris P. Kovatchev, PhD, head of computational neuroscience at the University of Virginia, Charlottesville, threw around unintelligible terms like "time-in-target traces," "control-variability grid analysis," and "Poincaré plots" with the comfort that other men use to discuss baseball statistics. With an Eastern European accent (he grew up in Rousse, Bulgaria), a trimmed goatee, and dark, deep-set eyes, he had the scary-smart look of a chess grandmaster. To make his point on the usefulness of computer models, he showed a slide of a flight simulator.

"Before complex machinery is put into use, simulators are really useful," he said. "Computer simulation can actually be more useful than an animal study. It can save many years and many experiments. Our simulator took a year to develop. It went to FDA. It was approved on January eighteenth of this year as an acceptable alternative to animal studies. We take a simulated patient, a simulated sensor, and a simulated pump. You can put in any control algorithm and see what happens. We have three hundred simulated subjects. Each one has twenty-six variables. A primary purpose of simulation is to test devices beyond the limits of their normal use, where failure is most likely. Do you live with someone who rolls over in bed thirty thousand times a night? You can do everything at the maximum rate and see what happens."

Francis J. Doyle III, PhD, who applies computer systems engineering principles to biological systems at the University of California, Santa Barbara, described how he uses simulations to control pumps on the fly. "We compare our representation of the patient to what the patient is actually doing," he said. "Feedback is now the difference between truth and my model of truth." A key to the approach, he said, is the use of a "moving horizon" in which the computer continuously projects what will happen, moment to moment, then continuously checks what does happen, moment to moment, and then continuously readjusts its forecast over and over again. "That's why it's often referred to as a moving horizon algorithm," Doyle said. "For those out there who play chess, this is the way Deep Blue did its chess calculations to beat Gary Kasparov. It forecasts far ahead; then when the opponent moves, it reforecasts."

After the math geeks had their say, skeptics spoke up from the audience. Tamborlane, for one, called the idea of using computer simulations instead of actual studies of living creatures "very unsettling."

"What are the criteria for judging the results of a simulated trial?" he asked.

Others jumped in with similarly leery questions, which the mathematicians tried their best to answer.

"It's perfectly fine to fail on the computer," Doyle said. "You can test your algorithm and beat up on it."

"We don't claim the simulators are like real life," Kovatchev said. "What we claim is—"

A persistent questioner cut him off, but Kovatchev fired back: "Will you let me finish my sentence?"

"I think there's a little tension in the room," said Kowalski, trying to calm things down. "One thing that should be clear is this is a tool. Simulators are just another option."

Stuart A. Weinzimer, MD, a colleague and collaborator of Tamborlane's at Yale, actually thanked Kovatchev for what he called his "ongoing mathematical education."

With curly black hair, olive skin, and heavy-lidded brown eyes, Weinzimer made for a striking visual foil to Tamborlane's more patrician bearing. Together, the pair had already published one of the first trials of a closed-loop system in humans. The blood-sugar levels of teens who controlled their own pumps, Weinzimer reported, were above 180 (considered moderately high) one-third of the time, and below 70 (the point where many people begin feeling the effects of a low sugar level) 9 percent of the time. By comparison, while on a closed-loop system being controlled by a computer, the same teens were above 180 only 15 percent of the time, below 70 only 3 percent of the time, and in the target zone a whopping 82 percent of the time. "That is our data," said Weinzimer, making the most eloquent case yet for the power of computers to beat human self-control.

Later in the afternoon, a session on the more practical, patient-oriented implications of an artificial pancreas was hosted by Kelly Close, the pixieish businesswoman who founded Close Concerns, an influential publisher of diabetes-related news for patients, manufacturers, and investors.

"I have been a patient with diabetes since I was a teenager," Close said. "For the decade before I got my pump in 1998, I was in the ER every six months on average [due to hypoglycemia]. When you recognize the paramedics in your ambulance, you know you have a problem. That's why, before continuous glucose monitoring was approved, my husband wouldn't let me travel alone." As investigators work toward an artificial pancreas, she said, "I don't think we should aim to get rid of all hypoglycemia. That will never happen. Let's just get rid of a lot of the hypoglycemia. Let's not let perfection be the enemy of the good."

Her first panelist, Tim Wysocki, PhD, chief of psychology and psychiatry at Nemours Children's Clinic in Jacksonville, Florida, explained why, no matter how good a closed-loop system might be, some people will never want it.

"Technology is all around us that makes the human condition better," he said. "Motorcycle helmets. Dog muzzles. Dental floss. Fire extinguishers. What do these technologies have in common? All are effective in countering or preventing adverse events. All are inexpensive and readily available. And none are used optimally. Will a closed-loop artificial pancreas be different? I don't think so."

The central problem, he said, is that some people, particularly adolescents, will see the devices as "controlling" them, and will resist. "Many patients will find the added responsibilities that comes with calibrating, safeguarding, maintaining, responding to alarms and false alarms, the possibility of pain or infection in the insertion sites—all of these kinds of things are more than some patients will be willing to tolerate."

At the final session of the day, representatives of the leading manufacturers of pumps and sensors, including Johnson & Johnson, DexCom, Abbott, Medtronic, Roche, Insulet, and Smiths Medical, tried to answer the questions of patients and researchers alike that they are taking too long to bring products to market.

"It all depends on you guys," Tamborlane told the panel. "I have this recurrent nightmare that we'll get this all worked out and then there will be fear from the corporate world in which the one patient dies in bed wearing a closed-loop system and you get a hundred-million-dollar lawsuit. Have you guys thought how you limit vulnerability to a lawsuit?"

John J. Mastrototaro, PhD, vice president of Global Medical, Scientific and Health Affairs at Medtronic Diabetes, compared the first step toward a fully automatic system to an automobile air bag.

In other words, just as an air bag inflates upon impact when it senses a crash, the computer would shut down the insulin pump automatically when it senses a dangerously low sugar level. "You're talking a fifty-to-one risk–benefit ratio," he said. "And the risk is mitigated by having the pump suspended only for a short period of time. The way we're proposing the introduction of the feature, it has mostly all upside and no downside."

But according to David L. Horwitz, MD, PhD, chief medical officer of the Johnson & Johnson Diabetes Institute, the risk of lawsuits is a legitimate concern. "Industry is willing to take a certain risk," he said, "but it's a question of what kind of constraints you can build around it. It becomes a public policy question as much as a corporate question."

"If you build an artificial pancreas that serves the needs of patients," said Larry Soler, vice president of government relations at the JDRF, "we will solve that problem. There is just no question in my mind that that problem will be solved. The focus of everyone on this panel should be on building the right product."

Asked by a doctor in the audience when the automatic shutoff of pumps in response to low sugar levels would be approved by the FDA, Soler went out on a limb and said 2011. "That's our goal," he said.

"For 2011, you'd need to be in Phase Three trials now," the audience member said.

And with a cryptic grin, Soler replied, "Maybe we are."

Plenty more went on the next day—presentations on the challenges of dealing with the sugar-lowering effects of exercise, which can last through the following night; on the annoying phenomenon of fibrous tissue fouling up the tip of glucose sensors, like leaves clogging a storm drain; and on the inevitability of sensors giving bad information, which programmers hope to thwart by mathematically detecting and correcting for them—but nothing that dissuaded me from the realization that the artificial pancreas is *this* close to reality.

Before heading back out into the inferno of the Washington Beltway in July, I attended a brief press conference following the meeting's conclusion, where JDRF officials spoke with excitement about the seven academic research centers they're funding around the world to push the artificial pancreas across the goal line. One reason for optimism, they said, is the growing consensus that the well-known inaccuracies of continuous sensors can be made up for with computer analysis.

"It's very hard to hit a hole in one from the tee," said Weinzimer, whose research with Tamborlane at Yale is funded in part by JDRF. "But if you make one small shot, make another shot, and in my particular case make twenty or thirty shots, you can get to the hole bit by bit."

"You're making up for inaccuracy with the continuous data," said Damiano.

"Frequency trumps accuracy," said Howard C. Zisser, MD, of Sansum Diabetes Research Institute in Santa Barbara.

"I believe in the next year that we'll demonstrate that people on these systems are much safer than people with traditional management," Kowalski said. "People with diabetes today are getting low virtually every single day and high virtually every single day. That puts them at risk. We have a technology that will help them. We just need to make sure it's safe."

"If I had diabetes," Weinzimer said, "I may or may not choose to wear a pump in the current open-loop iteration. I'd probably wear a sensor, but I don't know if I'd wear a pump. If I had a closed-loop system, even with current technology, I would absolutely wear it—absolutely. In a heartbeat."

I left that meeting in a state of rapture, certain that the holy grail was at last within reach.

INFINITE COMPLEXITY

Five months later, in December of 2008, the field was mired in bureaucratic hell. Only a single group in the United States was moving forward with a clinical trial of an artificial pancreas study in humans. The rest were all held up by continuing safety concerns from either the FDA or the device manufacturers. To top it off, I was still battling my insurance company, Oxford, just to get a continuous glucose monitor. After receiving my first rejection, back in September, I submitted a second lengthy application, including a letter from my doctor and readouts from my meter showing frequent, extreme highs and lows. Two weeks later, the second reply from Oxford stated: "Our medical director has determined that the request is denied because currently available evidence does not support the medical necessity of the continuous glucose monitoring system."

The one bright spot was that Boris Kovatchev, the Bulgarian with the goatee based at the University of Virginia, had agreed that I could participate in his clinical trial, as a test subject, as soon as it got back up and running, which was going to be in October. Which then was pushed to November. And then to January.

Finally, in anticipation of the trial going forward in the new year, I was asked to come in for a checkup and meeting with Kovatchev on December 10. The trial coordinator, Pam Mendosa, took a blood sample, weighed me, took my blood pressure, asked me what seemed like 5 billion questions, had me sign more forms than a mortgage application, and then sent me down the hall to meet with Kovatchev.

A Beethoven symphony played softly on his radio when I walked into his office, which was so spic-and-span it could have been mistaken for an IKEA display. A single folder lay open on his desk, and three patents were framed on the wall:

US 6,804,551 B2: Method and apparatus for the early diagnosis of subacute, potentially catastrophic illness. Issued October 12, 2004.

US 6,923,763 B1: Method and apparatus for predicting the risk of hypoglycemia. Issued August 2, 2005.

US 7,025,425 B2: Method, system, and computer program product for the evaluation of glycemic control in diabetes from self-monitoring data. Issued April 11, 2006.

Boris—I was calling him Boris now—wore a black North Face

vest, a blue work shirt, khaki pants, brown shoes, and tan socks. His fingers were stubby, his hazel eyes intense, his beard flecked with gray.

"The only active trial in the world now is ours," he said. "We tested the first four patients here earlier this year. They had practically no hypoglycemia at all. We will have twelve in all by the time we finish this first phase. You will be patient number nine."

I asked him why people remain so fearful of having a computer control their blood sugar, when computers already control everything from elevators to jet planes.

"I think people with diabetes are more easy to convince than the doctors," he replied. "The doctors tend to be more skeptical, because medicine has a long list of failures. If you put yourself in the place of an MD guy who treats diabetes and knows it's very difficult to control, and some engineer comes and says we're going to automate it and do better than you, that calls for suspicion. For doctors, the algorithm is a black box; they don't know what it's doing, and that increases the suspicion. And rightfully so. Until we prove in a clinical trial that it actually does better than ordinary control, we don't have a case.

"That's why our trial is constructed the way it is. Each patient goes through two identical days, separated by four weeks. The first day, the patient controls his blood glucose by the means he knows. The second day is our algorithm's control. We are hoping by comparing the first to the second day, we can do better than the patient. If we can show that, then we're okay. We'll publish it and hopefully it will be accepted as initial proof that we can do better with the computer."

Recollecting the comparison that Frank Doyle had made between the artificial pancreas's control algorithm and Deep Blue, I asked Boris which problem was harder to solve for a computer: maintaining a stable blood or beating a chess grandmaster.

"With chess you have a finite numbers of moves you can make," he answered. "The rules of the game are clear. The only question is how far ahead you can predict. Prediction horizon depends on the speed of the machine; it has to do several billion calculations. With diabetes control, the rules are clear somewhat—you know you have to keep blood sugar under control—but the number of moves are not finite, because the person's blood sugar changes constantly; it's infinitely complex. If you have exactly the same configuration on the chessboard and make a series of moves, Deep Blue will give you every time the same result. With diabetes it's not so. You know this yourself. If you have exactly the same breakfast today and tomorrow and inject exactly the same amount of insulin, the blood sugar you get will be different from day to day.

"If one could grasp the whole complexity of the human in real time," he continued, "then you would have perfect control of blood sugar. But that is not possible, because your complexity borders infinity. So we have to approximate the complexity. We do that with a model. The physician has in mind a certain model of his patient, given some characteristics, body weight, other things. That model is a simplification of the real patient by many orders of magnitude, and the physician has only occasional encounters with his or her patient, so adjustments in the control come a few months apart. When we do automated control, we also have a model of a patient, but it is based on sixteen variables, it is formulated to mathematical terms, and it readjusts frequently, in real time. It is still only an approximation of reality, but we believe it is a better approximation. At least, that's the claim."

Two things occurred to me. First, the best efforts of a person with diabetes to control his or her own blood sugar based on occasional finger pricks or even continuous glucose monitoring are doomed to failure. And second, by replacing our guesstimates and intuition with cold, hard calculations, the artificial pancreas would be like having a miniature Boris Kovatchev in our pocket.

Before leaving for his next appointment, Boris introduced me to Marc Breton, PhD, the systems engineer who was designing the software to control the artificial pancreas. I asked the young Frenchman whether an iPhone plug-in could be designed by some guy in a garage to control his own insulin pump based on continuous glucose monitoring.

"You could come up with a program of your own for your iPhone," he said. "But your iPhone can't talk to your sensor."

"I bet you could hack it," I said.

"I know you can hack it," he conceded. "But that would be illegal. You have to go through FDA. You cannot do it in a garage. And the information you would need on these devices is from manufacturers that are fairly secretive. These companies are in heavy competition between each other. The level of competition that exists in this field, between laboratories and companies, is insane. If you go to conferences, the ones we go to, we all talk about what we do, but at the same time we never tell anybody what we do. There is always the knowledge that you're not sharing all of what you know, and the person in front of you is not telling the whole story either. It's very strange. It's probably because this is a frontier, a border between academic science and industrial application."

Before leaving, I asked him why, from his perspective as a programmer, controlling blood sugar is so maddeningly complicated even though it involves just two variables, insulin and sugar level. Somehow he found the perfect metaphor to explain it: "The glucose you measure with a continuous glucose monitor was accurate fifteen minutes ago. The insulin you take does not start acting for twenty minutes, has a peak of action around forty-five minutes, and it continues to act for up to three hours. So you are acting on out-of-date data, and you're using a mode of action that will only kick in much later on. It's like you're driving a car down a winding road—but you aren't able to see that the road turned until you are fifteen yards past it, and turning the wheel will have no effect for two hundred yards more. If you're driving a car like that, you'd better have a good map."

PATIENT #109

Just over a month later, on January 14, 2009, I arrived back in Charlottesville to begin the first phase of my participation in Boris's trial, in which I would be controlling my own sugars while his computer observed and learned. At 9:30 P.M., Pam was waiting for me at their research office with Stacey Anderson, MD, the endocrinologist responsible for medical care in the study. They hooked me up to two Freestyle Navigator continuous glucose monitors—one on my left bicep, the other on my right—so that at least one would always be functioning for the study, in case the other went goofy. Each was labeled "109." That was my new identity: patient number 109, the ninth patient in the UVA study.

After getting hooked up, I went to the Red Roof Inn, where I would stay for the next day and a half, while the glucose monitors settled in, got calibrated, and were giving good numbers. That accomplished, I finally went to the UVA hospital at 4 P.M. on Friday, January 16, to meet Pam, Stacey, and a nurse named Wendie. Stacey taped an Omnipod pump onto the left side of my belly. Wendie then inserted an IV line onto my right forearm, so that they could begin drawing blood every 30 minutes. In all, I now had the pump, two continuous glucose monitors, and an IV line into my forearm. But then, to my surprise, they covered over the two Navigators so that I couldn't see their readings; their information would be transmitted wirelessly to Boris's computer, while I would have to make my decisions for how much insulin to take based only on my occasional finger-pricks with a hand-held meter.

Dinner at 6 P.M. was grilled salmon, rice, asparagus, Lorna Doone cookies, and a diet Sierra Mist with ice. I sat in the hospital bed watching the *NBC Nightly News, Wheel of Fortune,* a financial news show, a new episode of *Monk,* and a really bad John Wayne–Kirk Douglas movie from 1967. Around 9 P.M., I did a finger prick and found that my blood sugar was a bit high, at 190. My meter—which, like most meters today, comes with a simple program (a *very* simple program, using arithmetic that anyone could do on the back of an envelope) to suggest how much insulin to give—said I should take 2.5 units. I thought that was way too high, so I took just 1.5 units.

Around 11 P.M., I tested again and my sugar was now at 90. I knew I was heading low, so I walked out to the nurses' station, where Wendie was sitting. I told her I was going low and needed to turn off my basal insulin and eat something. But the study protocol, she said, required that I wait until my sugar actually went below 70 before I could take anything, and turning off the basal wasn't part of the protocol. I was struck by how strong the urge to eat something and follow my usual routine felt, as though my life depended on it—as if I really knew what the hell I was doing. Wendie decided to call Stacey, who also wanted me to stick to the protocol, but decided after much discussion that it would be okay if I ate something, although not to turn off the basal.

After all that, I decided to wait and follow their protocol, not wanting to screw up their study. An hour later, as I was trying to fall asleep, my sugar finally fell below 70. They gave me precisely four ounces of juice, for 15 grams of carbohydrate. I was sure that wouldn't be enough; normally I would have had at least twice that much juice and then a banana or piece of bread. (Although, in truth, normally the result would be that I'd wake up the next morning with a high of 240 or so.)

Now began Hell Night. A new nurse, who never introduced herself, showed up wearing a face mask because, she said, of a little cold. Once my sugar dropped below 70, she explained, the protocol required her to draw blood every 15 minutes until it returned to normal. But my sugar level didn't return to normal, as I had suspected it wouldn't. Instead, after more than an hour, it went low again. She gave me another juice. And kept coming in every 15 minutes to take blood, until finally, around 2:30 A.M., I was about ready to lose it and told the Masked Nurse, "This is crazy. I'm going to need some more food if it goes low again." But this time my sugars finally climbed up to the normal range, and she returned to testing my sugars "only" once every half hour.

The next morning, my sugar was near perfect, around 100. They gave me a can of Ensure for breakfast, as per their protocol. "Would you like vanilla or strawberry?" the nurse asked. I picked strawberry.

The can said it had 50 grams of carbo, and my meter told me that I should take 6.5 units of insulin.

By the time they were ready to give me lunch, around noon, my sugar had fallen to 53, low yet again. Here I was, a medical reporter writing a book about diabetes, sitting in a hospital, knowing exactly how many carbs I had eaten, following the advice of my nifty little meter, and still I had gone low not once, not twice, but three times! This was a tribute either to how incredibly stupid I really am or how ridiculously impossible this disease is to manage on one's own.

THE COMPUTER'S TURN

Four weeks later, on Friday, February 13, my date with destiny arrived. As before, I had to show up in Charlottesville two days early to have the pair of Freestyle Navigator CGMs attached to my arms; as before, I checked into the hospital at 4 P.M. on Friday to have the pump and IV line attached to my belly; as before, I was fed a meal of salmon, rice, asparagus, Lorna Doones, and diet Sierra Mist. But that is where the similarities to my prior visit ended.

This time, Marc Breton, the programmer, spent much of the night with me, hovering over his two Dell laptops, each attached to a cradle that held one of my CGM receivers, each one receiving data on my sugar level. Early on, he checked to see which of the two receivers was producing the more accurate data, decided it was the one on my left arm, and designated that one as the driver of the program that would control how much insulin I would get.

It turned out, however, that the FDA wasn't allowing the program to directly control my pump. Every 15 minutes, the program spit out a number saying how much insulin I needed; Stacey, the physician, had to read the number and make sure that it wasn't crazy; and then she would punch into a little hand-held device that same number to control the pump that actually delivered the insulin into me. The idea was that it added an extra layer of safety in case the program turned out to be a murderous version of Hal (the killer computer from *2001: A Space Odyssey*) or Skynet (the killer computer from the *Terminator* movies). Essentially, though, this would be a contest between me and Boris's computer, between man and machine.

At 10:15 P.M., with my sugar level at 125, the computer instructed Stacey to give me just 0.15 units. Not one unit; not half a unit . . . but fifteen-hundredths of a unit!

At 11:07 P.M., watching *Seinfeld,* I had a sudden urge to go running down the hall, skipping and yelling, in celebration of not having to worry about my insulin and sugar levels—of being, for one night only, magically freed of my diabetes. And then I felt myself close to tears, thinking what a pain in the ass, and how phenomenally distracting, it is to be constantly worrying about my goddamn sugars, instead of focusing on my work and my family and my friends and my life.

And so Friday the 13th gave way to Valentine's Day. During my previous stay at the hospital, in January, I had had two episodes of hypoglycemia overnight. This time I had none. In fact, throughout the night, my sugar level never went above 140 and never fell below 90. And the computer actually gave me far less insulin overnight than I would have given myself. From 9:30 on Friday night until 4:30 on Saturday morning, the program instructed Stacey to give me a total of just 2.3 units, compared to the 11 units that I had taken, following my standard basal rate, during the same overnight period in January. Less insulin, yet lower sugars overall? It seemed to make no sense.

"I think I can explain it," Boris told me on Saturday morning. "When people control their own insulin, they have many more hypoglycemic episodes. Hypoglycemia triggers counter-regulatory hormones that make your liver release glucose and build insulin resistance. That's why you need more insulin for the same job. One person in our study, his physician had him taking zero-point-six units of insulin per hour, and on that regimen he had four hypoglycemic events in one night, when brought here. When we put him on closed loop, he had no hypo-glycemia whatsoever, and for six hours overnight, the controller was saying he needed zero insulin. All that time his sugars stayed flat, between ninety and one hundred. Less insulin, fewer highs, and no lows. It's explainable, because when you get lows, you get a rebound."

He then informed me that between his site and his international collaborators' sites, in France and Italy, I was now the 20th patient in their study. "The largest study before now had only seventeen patients," he said. "So this is now the largest so far." Among the ten patients he personally had tested in Virginia, he said, there had been 17 lows while they were controlling their own sugars, and only two during closed-loop. "It's an eightfold reduction of hypoglycemia," he said.

With him that morning was Steven Patek, PhD, associate professor of systems and information engineering, who was working on improving their next generation of mathematical algorithm. The current algorithm, he said, wasn't so different from the calculus Isaac Newton invented to describe the motions of heavenly bodies.

"It's the same idea, the same kind of dynamical model for the glucose-insulin system," he said. "The forces are the insulin injections you take and the foods you eat. And these are pushing around the glucose concentration in your blood. It's called a deterministic linear model predictive control algorithm. But it's not really cognizant about noise in the system or uncertainty about parameter values. My specific work is to try to account for the uncertainties. We're not always certain about how much you eat or whether you eat; your glucose sensors also have inaccuracies. So what we have is imperfect knowledge. Instead of having truth, we have a noisy reflection of the truth. We as humans deal with uncertainty really well. My interest is in having our algorithm embrace that uncertainty."

After all the monitors and lines were removed from my body and the computers were packed up, I thanked Steve and Boris and Pam and Stacey and Marc and the nurses for all their fine work and returned to my diabetic world, in which the uncertainty embraces me. On Sunday morning, life was back to what passes for normal: my sugar was at 41 when I awoke, and then, after I overcompensated with a big breakfast, it climbed to 240 by noon. I felt like the cognitively challenged guy in the 1960s novel *Flowers for Algernon,* in which a drug temporarily makes him intellectually normal but then quickly wears off, leaving him challenged again. For 15 hours I was no longer diabetic. Now I was right back where I started.

Four months later, on June 6, 2009, Medtronic announced the first commercial realization of a semi-closed-loop system with the launch in Europe of an integrated pump and sensor with an automatic "low glucose suspend" feature that shuts off the pump when sugar levels are moving dangerously low. "We're making continued progress in our quest to fully automate diabetes management," said Chris O'Connell, a senior vice president at Medtronic. The company was reportedly in the process of submitting the automatic shutoff feature to the FDA for its approval and hoped to launch it in the United States by mid-2010.

Then again, all the plans of Medtronic and the other manufacturers just might be thrown out the window if a revolutionary new form of insulin now being tested by a Massachusetts biotechnology firm turns out to work as advertised. SmartInsulin, developed by Todd C. Zion, PhD, as part of his doctoral thesis in chemical engineering at the Massachusetts Institute of Technology, contains nanoparticles that chemically enclose insulin, releasing it into the bloodstream only when sugar levels rise. Injected once a day, SmartInsulin is designed to maintain normal sugar levels all on its own, kicking into action only when needed to avoid both highs and lows. Zion's firm, SmartCells, has so far received over $1.5 million in research funding from NIDDK and another $1 million from the JDRF. Should the firm succeed in bringing SmartInsulin to market, and if a single daily injection of it really maintains near-perfect sugar levels without the need for a pump, continuous glucose tester, or computer—well, then, the holy grail of an artificial pancreas will just have to collect dust in a showcase of obsolete diabetes technologies.

Either way, it sure will be nice going to sleep without worrying whether I'll wake up with my daughter spooning Marshmallow Fluff into my mouth—or whether I'll wake up at all.

CHAPTER 11

The Surgical Cure

Can Bariatric Surgery Stop Type 2 in Its Tracks?

N THE GREAT TRADITION of dorm-room cooking, there are those who settle for warming up a can of Chef Boy-R-Dee, and then there is Tom Pallozzi-Haynes. As a student in the 1980s at William Paterson College in Wayne, New Jersey, he liked to throw together a gourmet meal of braciola (pronounced, Jersey style, as *braz-shule*), thin slices of rolled-up veal filled with prosciutto and cheese, slow-cooked to perfection in a zesty Italian gravy. On his dorm-room hot plate.

"You have a gift," one of his buddies told him on a Sunday evening, after he had made dinner for the usual group. "You should think about becoming a chef."

A light bulb switched on over Tom's head. His grandparents had been paying for his college education, but since the age of 13 he had worked in the food-service business, first as a dishwasher at a German restaurant in his hometown of Bloomingdale, New Jersey, then at his parents' deli and catering business in Paterson. He decided to quit college and follow his passion. After working his way through the New York Culinary School, he graduated first in his class and was hired as an apprentice at the famed Plaza Hotel in New York City.

By 1992, at the age of 25, Tom had worked his way up to become the chef at the Plaza's Oyster Bar restaurant. He turned out to be such a fast oyster-shucker that he was selected as the U.S. representative in the world oyster-shucking competition, in Finland.

"I want to win! I'm going to win," he told a reporter for the Associated Press, punching the air. "Yes!"

Donald Trump, then owner of the Plaza, sent his corporate helicopter to transport Tom to the airport. Once in Finland, Tom later told the *Record,* "I expected to play in the Little League finals, but it was the World Series. It was the Olympics of oysters." Actually, it was the fifth annual World Championship Oyster Grand Prix. Tom shucked 30 oysters in two minutes and 19 seconds, good enough for third place.

Soon he was an executive chef at the Plaza, participating in celebrity events and living large. A little too large. By 1999, the energetic, driven young man was diagnosed with type 2 diabetes. He tried Weight Watchers, the Atkins diet, anything that seemed promising. His weight inched past 250, fell back down to 210, and then began the return trip. Even when eating little but meat and avoiding all carbohydrate ("I'm a meatatarian," he liked to joke), his sugars remained high. He went on Byetta injections for a while, which helped him lose weight, but when the FDA issued a warning in 2007 that the drug might be linked to an increased risk of acute pancreatitis, his doctor ran the recommended blood test, found worrisome signs, and took him off it. By 2008, Tom's primary-care doctor had him taking two of the more popular brand-name drugs for type 2: Amaryl (one of the new, longer-acting sulfonylureas) and Glucophage (metformin). With a demanding new job as senior associate director of admissions at the Institute of Culinary Education in New York, he found food to be the only thing that kept his energy level up. Married, with a newborn son, he had trouble walking more than a single flight of stairs. Just 41 years old, Tom could see the writing on the wall: his health was spiraling downward despite the best that pharmaceutical treatment of diabetes could offer.

Then, on April 20, 2008, he caught a *60 Minutes* episode about the diabetes-relieving effects of gastric bypass surgery. Although the highly respected show had an unfortunate history of making much ado about dubious medical "breakthroughs"—like shark cartilage (supposedly a cure for cancer) and *hoodia gordonii* (claimed to help with weight loss)—this one was backed by impressive scientific evidence. Correspondent Lesley Stahl cited studies claiming that 80 percent of diabetics come off all their medications following bariatric surgery, even before losing much of their weight.

Stahl introduced viewers to Italian surgeon Francesco Rubino, MD, who had become curious about why the surgery worked so quickly to relieve diabetes. In experiments with diabetic rats, Rubino found that even without constricting their stomachs, he could make their diabetes disappear just by rerouting the plumbing of their small intestines to go around the upper portion, called the duodenum. Then, if he reattached the duodenum, the diabetes returned. "This meant diabetes could essentially be removed with a scalpel," Stahl said. She interviewed other doctors who shared that view, and presented a panel of patients who said their bariatric surgeries had cured their diabetes in days or weeks. "I went into the hospital on Friday, came home on Monday, and dumped my pills," said one.

Impressed, Tom contacted Rubino, who had just taken a new job in the United States as director of gastrointestinal metabolic surgery at New York Presbyterian/Weill Cornell Medical Center. Unable to perform surgery in the United States until passing U.S. medical licensing tests, however, Rubino referred Tom in the meanwhile to the endocrinologist in his practice. She brought Tom in for testing and discovered his A1C to be over 10—dangerously elevated, compared to a normal level of less than 6. She took him off Amaryl, kept him on Glucophage, and started him on insulin. Soon he was up to 50 units of long-acting

Lantus insulin in the evening (to control his overnight blood-sugar levels), 20 more units of Lantus in the morning, and 17 units (or more) of short-acting Novolog insulin with every meal. His weight climbed due to the insulin, but as spring turned to summer and summer to fall, he just kept waiting for Rubino's license to come through.

THE LOWER INTESTINAL THEORY

The evidence in favor of bariatric surgery as a treatment for type 2 diabetes, while not nearly as strong as some would like, is nevertheless compelling and consistent. One of the most startling reports, published in 2007 in the *New England Journal of Medicine*, compared the risk of death among 7,925 people who underwent gastric bypass surgery against 7,925 people who, according to their driver's license application, were severely obese. After just over seven years, those who underwent the gastric bypass were 40 percent less likely to die than those who did not have the surgery. The risk of dying specifically because of diabetes, the researchers found, was 92 percent lower among those who underwent the surgery. Death from cancer and heart disease was also significantly lower following surgery (although deaths due to accidents or suicides were, strangely, higher).

In January of 2008, Australian researchers published a randomized trial in the *Journal of the American Medical Association*, involving 55 obese patients who were assigned to receive either adjustable gastric banding or conventional medical treatment. After two years, complete remission of diabetes was seen in 22 of the people who underwent banding (73 percent), compared to only four (13 percent) in the conventional-therapy group—meaning that surgery proved more than five times better at relieving diabetes during the two years of the study.

The results were impressive enough to draw an editorial in the *New York Times*. "Evidence is accumulating that the best treatment for type 2 diabetes related to obesity may well be the most drastic:

stomach-shrinking surgery, perhaps accompanied by intestinal rearrangements," the editorial stated. "That such extreme remedies would even be considered is a measure of how intractable the intertwined epidemics of obesity and diabetes have become in the United States."

Even more recently, in March of 2009, the *American Journal of Medicine* published a "meta-analysis" analyzing 621 prior studies involving a total of 135,246 patients. The analysis found that 78.1 percent of diabetic patients who underwent bariatric surgery had been effectively cured of their diabetes, requiring no further medication, and that 86.6 percent saw at least some improvement of their diabetic symptoms.

Despite such results, many endocrinologists who have devoted years to treating diabetes with diet, exercise, and medications insist that much longer, much larger, multi-center trials are necessary to prove the benefits of surgery.

"You need to follow them not for two years, but for ten and fifteen years," said F. Xavier Pi-Sunyer, MD, past president of the American Diabetes Association, when I asked him about surgery.

Surgeons like Rubino, however, believe that the results seen with gastric banding or stomach stapling are mild compared to what can be achieved with the right technique. Banding and stapling, after all, merely make the stomach smaller, forcing people to eat less. A far more powerful effect, however, has been seen with techniques that move the lower portion of the small intestine up higher in the tract, so that the stomach empties into it directly. It turns out that this lower portion of the small intestine releases a variety of potent, glucose-lowering hormones when exposed to food—including GLP-1, the same hormone that a popular, injected drug for type 2, Byetta, seeks to mimic. What's more, the upper portion of the small intestine—the duodenum and jejunum—appears to release hormones that might actually make diabetes worse. By putting the duodenum and jejunum to rest, then, while moving up the lower intestine, the intestines are ideally repositioned to produce the hormones most conducive to avoiding diabetes. At least, so goes the "lower intestinal theory."

But it's not only surgeons who are beginning to see the actions of the lower intestine as fundamental to the development of type 2 diabetes. In the view of David Cummings, MD, associate professor of medicine and deputy director of the Diabetes Endocrinology Research Unit at the University of Washington in Seattle, "There is a great deal of evidence for something special going on in the lower intestine that has a unique effect on blood sugars."

Evidence in support of the lower intestinal theory has been accumulating quickly in human clinical trials. A 2007 paper by Judith Korner, MD, PhD, assistant professor of clinical medicine and director of the Weight Control Center at Columbia University, found increased levels of GLP-1, and lower insulin levels, in 13 patients who underwent a Roux-En-Y procedure (in which most of the stomach is stapled off, and the remaining part is rerouted directly to the lower portion of the small intestine), but not in ten patients who had gastric banding.

Fundamental to the notion of surgery for type 2 diabetes is that it should work in people who are not extremely obese, the usual candidates for stomach surgery. The standard measure of who is or isn't overweight or obese, the body mass index, accounts for both height and weight. A 2008 paper by Wei-Jei Lee, MD, of National Taiwan University compared 44 patients with a BMI below 35 (the minimal level at which most insurance companies will consider paying for bariatric surgery) to 157 patients with a higher BMI. A year after surgery, 89.5 percent of the thinner patients had normal blood sugars, compared to 98.5 percent of the others. The surgery, Lee concluded, worked only slightly less well in the lighter patients to relieve their diabetes.

But with only an estimated 1 percent of morbidly obese patients undergoing bariatric surgery as it is, in part because of its expense, researchers are investigating the possibility of gaining its benefits without making a single incision. Lee Kaplan, MD, PhD, associate professor of medicine and associate chief of research in the division of gastroenterology at Harvard Medical School, recently described his research with the EndoBarrier gastrointestinal liner—an impermeable device implanted in the upper intestine, like a garbage bag liner, via the mouth, to block absorption of nutrients. By blocking the uppermost part of the small intestine, it permits nutrients to flow directly to the lower portion without being absorbed. He studied 19 patients with type 2, who either received the liner or underwent a sham endoscopy, with no liner inserted. Twelve weeks after implantation, patients who received the liner experienced "a significant decrease in A1C," he said, compared to patients who underwent the sham procedure. "By thirty weeks, there was a 2.9 percent decrease of A1C on average."

Because it can be inserted or removed during an outpatient procedure in a surgeon's office, the device holds out the promise of extending the diabetes-relieving surgery to large numbers of people with type 2. But since it is not yet approved by the FDA, for now people like Tom Pallozzi-Haynes must rely on more traditional bariatric procedures if they choose to go the surgical route.

EAT HEAVY

Two days before he was finally scheduled to go under the knife, I met Tom at the Tick Tock Diner in Clifton, New Jersey. As legions of classic diner fans know, the Tick Tock has a two-word motto, emblazoned in neon over its gleaming chrome roof for drivers passing by on Route 3: "Eat Heavy."

He was already seated in a booth, drinking an iced tea, when I joined him. With a shaved head, piercing blue eyes, and the rather round face one would expect of a 272-pound man, he reminded me a bit of "Curly" from the old *Three Stooges* movies, only smarter and better-looking.

"Are you guys okay now?" asked the big-haired waitress after I sat down.

"I'm good for now," Tom told her. "I'm on clear liquids for the next forty-eight hours."

"Really?" she said. "Wow."

I ordered coffee and asked Tom if he didn't feel a bit crazy for undergoing surgery in order to treat his diabetes.

"One of my biggest frustrations being diabetic," he said, "is all the people who say to me, 'If you just eat broccoli, it will go away.' I'm a chef by trade. I've been around food for over twenty years. My wife's family will say, 'Oh, it's your diet, it's your diet.' I've tried all kinds of diets. I have the dearest, most loving wife who subscribes to every medical newsletter out there. 'Take this vitamin, take that supplement,' Sophy tells me. It doesn't work. What people don't realize is diabetes is a disease. I've had it for ten years now. This is the best chance of recovery for me, and having better function of my pancreas. This is going to take a lot of stress off my heart, my pancreas, my liver, my blood pressure."

He and Dr. Rubino had decided together that the best procedure for him would be the Roux-En-Y, to not only shrink down his stomach, but also get the benefit of rerouting his intestine to bypass the duodenum and jejunum.

"I'll be eating a lot less," Tom said. "My diet is going to be very, very restrictive. Being a chef who loves food, it's going to be a major, major challenge. It's going to be a whole new lifestyle for me."

I asked whether he was doing it primarily to lose weight, to relieve his diabetes, or both.

"I'm absolutely doing it for the diabetes," he said. Then he thought a moment and said, "It's not about me anymore, it's about my son. Sebastian is just two. To see him play football in high school, play soccer with him and be around for that . . . Without this surgery, my diabetes is just going to continue to spiral downward."

I asked him whether he was at all nervous about the procedure.

"My biggest curiosity is what I'm going to feel like after," he said. "Am

I going to feel hypoglycemic? Am I going to be hungry all the time? That's my biggest concern, how my chemistry will adjust."

Two days later, shortly before 8 A.M. on Thursday, April 16, 2009, I met Lezlie Greenberg, a press liaison for New York Presbyterian/Weill Cornell Medical Center, in the lobby at 525 East 68th Street. Up on the surgical floor, both of us changed into blue gowns, with booties and white face masks, before being allowed into the surgical suite where Tom was already anesthetized. With his legs spread-eagled so that Dr. Rubino could stand between them perched on a four-inch-high stool, Tom was draped in sheeting that covered everything except an 18-inch square over his ample stomach.

"Time-out," said a nurse, Lola, at 8:20 A.M., as part of their standard procedure to be sure they were doing the correct operation on the correct patient. Two other nurses, a medical student, a surgical fellow, and an anesthesiologist completed the cast in the operating theater.

And then it began. The operation would be a minimally invasive laparoscopic procedure, with four knitting-needle-like probes quickly jabbed through Tom's abdomen. The first of the probes was a tiny video camera. Looking up at the 28-inch-wide, high-definition, flat-screen monitor hanging over Tom's head, I saw the image go from a view of the room to yellow, squiggly, tangled stuff surrounded by tiny red blood vessels. As Dr. Rubino manipulated two of the probes, he stared at the television monitor as if conducting simulated surgery on a Wii.

Blobs of yellow fat passed across the screen until the pink sausage of the intestine came into view. Using a mark on the end of his grasping device like a yardstick to measure distances, Dr. Rubino reached his destination. He switched from a grasper to a cutting device, and I could hear a stapler-like clicking as he clipped off the intestine just below the jejunum. At least, that's what he said he was cutting; it might as well have been poor Tom's liver for all I could tell.

"It's not as complicated as it looks," Dr. Rubino tried to assure me.

I laughed and said, "No, I think it *is* as complicated as it looks."

Measuring up toward the stomach, Dr. Rubino then cut another portion.

"What happens to the rest of the intestine that you went around?" I asked him.

"We just leave it," he said. "It has a blood supply. It will drip a little bile. Otherwise it just remains there."

It seemed bizarre, but then, what's not bizarre about mucking around inside a man's intestines?

At 9:15 Dr. Rubino began cutting into the stomach, which looked to me like a pale, pink ham swaddled in a blanket of orange marmalade. The ultrasound shears cut and coagulated blood simultaneously, and wisps of smoke swirled into the picture on the television.

By 9:25 he was done making a small pouch from the once-large stomach and was ready to connect the top of the intestine to the lower end. He clasped the two ends, tugged them toward each other, then inserted a special device that somehow stapled them together from the inside. At 9:58 he was sewing the newly joined intestine to the tissue surrounding it with tight, tiny loops that would shame a seamstress.

At 10:42 the video camera was pulled out and Dr. Rubino headed into the hall, leaving the closing of the incisions to the surgical fellow. I asked him how patients like Tom deal with hunger following surgery.

"This is what's fantastic about the operation," he told me in the hallway, lined with windows offering a spectacular view of the East River. "The hunger is gone. That's why patients who try to lose weight fail—they feel so hungry. That's the powerful effect of the hormones coming from the duodenum."

If Dr. Rubino's lower-intestine theory is correct, I realized, the gut hormones act like a thermostat in a home, switching on hunger when they sense that a precious pound or two of weight have been lost. In obese people, their thermostat is simply set on high, and hormones signaling hunger are released even though they're 100 pounds overweight. By rerouting the intestines, Dr. Rubino is dialing down the thermostat.

THE SHOWDOWN:
SURGEONS VERSUS ENDOCRINOLOGISTS

To some, the idea of "curing" diabetes with bariatric surgery is seen as a cop-out or worse—a moral failure by patients and an exploitative farce by surgeons, as preposterous as "curing" a headache with a guillotine. This disdain for a surgical solution was on display at an international meeting Rubino organized the autumn before he performed Tom's surgery, while still awaiting his medical license. Planned with the best of intentions, the First World Congress on Interventional Therapies for Type 2 Diabetes, held at the New York Marriott Marquis Hotel on September 15 and 16, 2008, proved to be a cantankerous battleground of surgeons, medical doctors, and public health officials defending turf and tossing scientific turd bombs. I loved it. Watching doctors fight is more entertaining than pro wrestling.

Things started out nicely enough. Richard Daines, MD, commissioner of health for New York State, told about his 20-year experience conducting physicals at a Boy Scouts camp each summer. "Before my eyes I saw this epidemic occur, with more and more boys overweight and obese," he said. "Toward the end I saw the first of these boys actually come in with type 2 diabetes." He called the surgical treatment of diabetes an "outside-the-box, perhaps revolutionary approach. We know the interventional approach will be important; we don't know how important. We know there are benefits; we don't know how many risks."

The Congress was then officially opened by José Ángel Córdova Villalobos, MD, Mexico's minister of health. "More than twenty-six percent of our children under ten are obese or overweight," he told the hundreds of attendees. "The first cause of death in Mexico is now diabetes. It's very exciting to learn about the new possibilities with surgery."

Rubino then took the stage to explain why he had organized the Congress. Of average height, with thinning black hair and a soft voice, he could not be called an imposing figure. And yet he had a gentle, reassuring relentlessness about him, working slowly to immobilize his critics like molasses engulfing a fly.

"Diabetes has become one of the most common diseases in the world," he began. "It is the single greatest emerging threat to public health. Yet with current medical therapies, it is rarely forced into remission, and usually comes at the expense of continuing effort and treatment. Surgery offers the promise of endurable remission with a single procedure, once in a lifetime. It is something we have never seen in the history of diabetes. It questions the definition of diabetes as a chronic, progressive, irreversible illness. It forces the question for the first time: can we go beyond treating diabetes, to curing it? We can't claim it's a cure yet, because we don't know the cause of diabetes, and therefore we can't say if we are eradicating that cause. But ninety-two percent of patients saw their diabetes relieved following surgery in a recent *New England Journal of Medicine* study."

A disarmingly savvy speechmaker, Rubino took a page from the Obama playbook by laying out the two opposing camps, for and against surgery, and then recontextualizing the debate as a false dichotomy, in the process placing himself above the fray.

"At the beginning of a new practice," he said, "most people have the tendency to think in terms of black and white. My own opinion is that surgery will never be the first line of treatment for diabetes. Surgery is almost never the first line of treatment for any disease, even those conventionally thought to be surgical. If you have gallstones, coronary stenosis, you try medical treatments first.

"Bariatric surgery," he continued, "is often characterized as a radical, potentially lethal surgery. Compared to other surgeries, its risk is lower than many others, as low as hip replacement. Yet no other elective surgery generates so much concern and fear. The mortality rate from bariatric surgery is three-tenths of one percent."

Now, having prepped his patients, as it were, he cut to the quick with a surgeon's precision.

"Some assume that bariatric surgery is appropriate only for the obese," he said. "Yet there are obese people who have normal sugars, and people with normal weight who have type two diabetes and all the associated risk factors for mortality. At this point we should question whether or not weight is the most important thing, or whether body weight may be just a surrogate of a metabolic alteration that links diabetes to obesity. It might not be weight per se that causes diabetes."

A growing body of research, he said, shows that the GI tract may have the most critical influence on type 2 diabetes of any organ in the body—more so than the insulin-releasing pancreas, the sugar-storing liver, or even the fat cells.

"The conventional paradigm of type two doesn't take the GI tract into consideration," Rubino said. "We have been too focused on the microscopic level; we have missed the big picture. Surgery might actually be fixing what is broken. If this is true, it has something to do with the small intestine. The most effective operations are those that actually put a large segment of the intestine at rest, completely and definitively. It is a provocative and inflammatory hypothesis, but it is an example of what is at stake here. A cure for diabetes may be possible in our lifetime."

Game on.

It was now the establishment's turn to defend the status quo and put the upstart surgeons in their place.

"Nationwide, the proportion of people with diabetes achieving good control is increasing," said the president of the American Diabetes Association, John Buse, MD, chief of endocrinology at the University of North Carolina in Chapel Hill. "About fifty-five percent of people in the U.S. with diabetes have an A1C of less than seven, and the average is 7.2. That's a dramatic improvement over the last decade. Part of this is because we're making the diagnosis earlier, but even on patients on insulin and oral agents, there has been an improvement. We have entered an era with new and exciting medical therapies."

Allison Goldfine, MD, associate professor of medicine at Harvard

Medical School and head of the section of clinical research at the Joslin Diabetes Center, described some rare but extremely serious cases of diabetics who, following bariatric surgery, had the opposite problem, of extreme low sugars, so persistent that a few even had to have their pancreas removed. "Some of these cases develop five to ten years after the bariatric procedure," she noted.

Concerns such as these provoked a word of caution from the surgeon whose 1995 paper in the *Annals of Surgery* is considered by many to have touched off the modern movement to treat diabetes with the scalpel rather than the syringe.

"Our first responsibility is the protection of the public," said Walter J. Pories, MD, professor of surgery and deputy director of the Metabolic Institute for the Study of Diabetes and Obesity at East Carolina University in Greenville, North Carolina. For all the promise of bariatric surgery as a treatment for diabetes, he said, "Since both the medical advances and the surgical results appear so promising and since diabetes is exploding, we owe it to our patients to find answers as quickly as possible through fair, prospective national studies."

A middle ground was staked out by Bernie Zinman, MD, a colleague of Dosch's at the University of Toronto and one of the most highly respected diabetes researchers in the world.

"You don't always need randomized controlled trials to draw a conclusion," he said. "The best example of that is smoking. There are no randomized controlled trials of the effect of smoking on cardiovascular outcome. Such a trial would be unethical. I would argue that for someone with a BMI over forty-five [considered "morbidly" obese by physicians], who has sleep apnea, diabetes, and difficulty just getting around—I don't think anyone questions that in such a case, bariatric surgery can be helpful. What we're discussing here is for patients under BMI of thirty-five whose diabetes can be treated; they may need insulin or they may not. In that circumstance, what we need is clear data from randomized trials. There is tremendous bias from small series from surgeons who are highly motivated to show a response."

Finally, it was time for the surgeons to make their move. While taking the knife to the bowels of a person with a BMI of 35 or greater had been endorsed by an NIH consensus conference back in 1991, the question now was whether the surgery could be recommended for treating diabetes per se, and in people whose BMI is under 35. With representatives from leading medical organizations seated at a long table on the stage, the case for surgery was pressed by moderator Phil Schauer, MD, past president of the American Society for Metabolic and Bariatric Surgery and director of the Cleveland Clinic Bariatric and Metabolic Institute.

"We enthusiastically endorse continued research," said Jeffrey Mechanick, MD, a member of the board of directors of the American Association of Clinical Endocrinologists. "However, anything outside the framework of research, we as a society are not able to endorse at this time. It's really the lack of sufficient long-term data related to the benefits and mainly the risks of these procedures. We live in an incomplete world. We can't wait for complete knowledge to make all our decisions. But at the present time, today, while I'm speaking, we're unable to endorse setting guidelines, saying when we would recommend a surgical procedure specifically for diabetes."

Like a debate club competitor, Schauer tried to catch Mechanick in a logical inconsistency. "Are you saying you wouldn't endorse the 1991 NIH guidelines, which supported surgery for diabetes in people with a BMI of thirty-five or greater?"

"It's a matter of semantics," parried Mechanick. "We would endorse surgery for obesity with other co-morbidities, which may be diabetes. The issue is, would you recommend surgery specifically for type two diabetes, when BMI happens to be thirty-five or over?"

"So you're saying you need randomized evidence for type two diabetes, but not for obesity?"

Rubino tried to get between the disputants. "I'm afraid there's a misunderstanding when we talk about these things," he said. "To say that surgery may be indicated at a certain BMI, that is not an endorsement as a first-line treatment. We're saying that if the patient with diabetes has no other option, it shouldn't be the BMI to discriminate over who can get this. There's no evidence that if you select a specific BMI cutoff, you can tell me which patient with diabetes will benefit from the surgery."

"That consensus statement on obesity from 1991 was based on much lower evidence," added Schauer, addressing Mechanick with all the diplomacy of a prosecutor at a war-crimes tribunal, "yet you fully endorse that concept. But when you bring in diabetes, you're requiring a different level of evidence."

"Surely you're not suggesting that every seventeen years we shouldn't mature with our understanding of evidence-based medicine?" Mechanick replied, his voice betraying obvious frustration. "We have more sophisticated methods for understanding medicine today. I do think there is a place for demanding more rigor."

Next up in the gladiatorial ring was Sue Kirkman, MD, vice president for clinical affairs of the ADA. Wearing a demure white sweater to offset her black dress, short black hair, and black-framed glasses, she voiced a view as conservative as her style, offset by a welcomed note of self-deprecating humor. She emphasized that the association would be issuing new guidelines in 2009 recognizing the value of bariatric surgery for people with diabetes uncontrolled by medical therapy and a BMI of at least 35. But going under the 35 barrier, she said, was something the organization believed to be not yet supported by sufficient evidence.

"Yes, we as an association are conservative, we are slow to change," said Kirkman. "We require high levels of evidence. I know that frustrates people. I figure that if we have people on all sides annoyed with us, we must be doing the right thing."

Next on the firing line was Gojka Roglic, MD, a thin woman (but then, remarkably, not a single participant at the meeting appeared to be overweight) who hailed from the former Yugoslavia and now represented the World Health Organization on diabetes.

"I suspect the World Health Organization might be even more conservative than the ADA," Roglic said. "We have to satisfy a much larger clientele than the population of the USA. We are responsible for poor and middle-income countries as well as wealthier ones, and they are struggling with the management of diabetes in primary care, with people having to go long distances, inadequately trained personnel, the unavailability of medication. We cannot even translate the science of what has already been proven to work in diabetes. What will happen is that rich people in poor countries will continue to do what they do now: they will go to the United States for treatment."

Then came George Alberti, MD, an endocrinologist at the University of Newcastle in England and representative of Diabetes UK, the British version of the ADA. "There is probably no bariatric surgery being done in England for the primary purpose of diabetes," he said. "It should be done purely in the context of clinical trials."

At last, one endocrinologist spoke up in favor of surgery, even taking his fellow physicians to task for refusing to acknowledge the benefits of surgery. "This is not a turf battle, this is not a matter of stealing patients from endocrinologists," said David Cummings, MD, associate professor of medicine and deputy director of the Diabetes Endocrinology Research Unit at the University of Washington in Seattle.

Schauer drove home the point. "It's not us versus you; we're all physicians seeking the best care of our patients," he said. "Why don't you work with us to convince the NIH to support the randomized trials you want? We need to all work together."

Even Rubino made a final gambit, suggesting to the endocrinologists that endorsing reasonable guidelines now could forestall more radical procedures by surgeons later. "That is why we need today, and not tomorrow, to establish widely accepted clinical guidelines, to make sure that we promote respect of safe standards."

But the endocrinologists were having none of it.

"There is suggestive early data that bariatric surgery for diabetes may be of value," conceded Harold Lebovitz, MD, professor of medicine in the division of endocrinology and metabolism/diabetes at the State University of New York Health Sciences Center in Staten Island. "But until the randomized studies are done comparing surgery to best medical care, the argument will go on between you and us."

As the Congress came to an end, the wait-for-more-data school plainly did not satisfy the surgeons. "I'm just worried we are procrastinating on finding the absolute ideal mechanism of action before we go in and encourage surgery," said Tessa van der Merwe, MB, ChB, PhD, director of Netcare Bariatric Centres of Excellence in Parktown, South Africa. "I'm concerned that we're waiting for that one ideal trial that is going to come around in ten years and provide us with all the data."

In the hallways and aisles of the dispersing meeting, the endocrinologists were livid over having been pressed so hard to support guidelines in favor of surgery.

"Schauer was so unfair, so unfair," grumbled a prominent physician. "And Cummings was almost as bad."

"I was on the verge of telling Schauer that a moderator should not be taking a point of view and pounding away at people who disagree," said another top diabetologist.

Like I said, it was one heck of a good show.

NO NEEDLES, NO PILLS

Eight days after his surgery, Tom was already off both of the pills he had been taking for diabetes, Glucophage and Amaryl, and was down from taking 70 units of long-acting insulin per day (to cover between-meal sugar levels) to just 25 units. "I'm supposed to take the Novolog [short-acting] insulin if my sugar goes above two hundred, but I haven't had any readings yet where I needed to inject it," he told me by telephone from his home.

He had had some pain when he awoke from the surgery, from the air they inject into the bowels to keep them as wide-open as possible.

"Getting that air out of you takes a while," he said. "You basically pass gas is how it gets out of you. It never felt so good to break wind in my life."

With just a bit of lingering stiffness and achiness, he said, he basically felt fine.

One thing he had already noticed was a lack of the food cravings that had always bedeviled him. "Definitely my appetite is changed," he said. "I had Cream of Wheat for breakfast yesterday. One little packet, I was good. I used to eat the whole box."

A month and a half later, on June 10, we spoke again. This time he was driving from work to his home in eastern Pennsylvania.

"I'm off all my meds," Tom said. "I'm down fifty-three pounds, to two-twenty. No needles, no pills."

I asked the "meatatarian" whether he was able to eat any steak yet. "I'm eating flounder, dark-meat chicken, soft vegetables, cereal, poached eggs, protein shakes. I can't eat a steak yet. Learning how to eat is a learning process. I used to eat a pound of pasta; that's a physical impossibility now."

And how about those hunger pangs?

"I don't have any hunger," he said. "I don't have a sense like I want to go eat and snack on something. I have to press myself to eat during the day. I used to sit down and eat a nice pint of Ben & Jerry's with chocolate syrup and not think anything of it. My breakfast now is two or three poached eggs with some white toast, maybe a slice—that's it. Before I could sit and eat a pancake breakfast with home fries, bacon, and toast. I can't do that anymore, and I don't even crave it."

Did he think there might be a bit of self-hypnosis hocus-pocus going on, and that eventually the cravings would return?

"I think there's definitely a chemical change that occurred," he said. "It is definitely dramatically different. I used to come out of work, I would stop at this Chinese restaurant in Denville. I'd want some shrimp toast and egg-drop soup and a double order of shrimp and garlic sauce. I have no desire to do it now. I used to go downstairs for lunch at the Outback and have a cheeseburger. Now I don't even want to. I have to remind myself to have a shake. It's really a significant difference. I used to dread having to walk up stairs. I'm on the sixth floor. I'm walking up and down and it doesn't faze me. Fifty-three pounds off your legs and knees make a big, big difference."

Wasn't it a bit surreal, I asked him, to no longer have the same urge to eat that he had before the surgery?

"It is surreal," he conceded. "But in a good way. Before I was a slave to the medication and a slave to food for energy. I knew I was spiraling downward. Not having to take medications, it's a good thing. Am I missing to have a cut of Grade-eight Wagyu? Sure."

Being a vegetarian, I had no idea what "Grade-eight Wagyu" is, and told him so.

"It's a Japanese beef," he said. "Good stuff. Sure I miss it. You remember the flavor of something like that. But I'm not craving it from an addiction. It's really different. That was my big concern: was I going to be starving and not able to eat? That's not been the case. I'm eating about 750 calories per day for now, and I'm more than full. I used to eat 3,700 calories a day, if not more. I have a lot more energy, I can tell you that. And I'm able to get into my nice clothes again."

Tom's surgery to cure his type 2, I realized, was not unlike the artificial pancreas to cure type 1. Neither is elegant or natural; both have their drawbacks—and both are expensive. But by golly, they work. Which is, of course, a huge first in the history of diabetes. And pondering the surreal effectiveness of Tom's surgery made me think back to Logan County, West Virginia. How much better off would Randy Blankenship and his ten brothers and sisters have been, I wondered, if they could have received bariatric surgery to cure their diabetes 20 years ago, rather than putting up with a lifetime of medications that never cured anything?

Of course, Dr. Rubino has not yet proved that bariatric surgery will permanently cure type 2. Perhaps Tom's diabetes will eventually return one day. And certainly the artificial pancreas is no match for a working natural pancreas; it might be close to a cure, practically speaking, but not biologically. The real, honest-to-God Cure with a capital C—the kind that doesn't require costly surgery or high-tech gadgets but can be delivered with, say, a few weeks of pills and then, *poof!* you're all better—that is what will win somebody a Nobel Prize one day. But when? Could it possibly be in our lifetimes? Is waiting for a real cure like waiting for Godot? To find out, I headed west to San Francisco, to meet the one researcher described by colleagues and competitors alike to be as close as anyone has ever been to achieving the great dream of curing type 1 diabetes.

CHAPTER 12

The Biological Cure

*The Search for a Pill that Cures Type 1,
Once and for All*

"WE SHOULD SAY CLEARLY and at the outset, this is a study of mice, but it's generating excitement because it could hold the key to putting diabetes patients into a kind of permanent remission."

So Brian Williams, host of the *NBC Nightly News,* introduced the latest bulletin from the front lines of biological research into curing diabetes the old-fashioned way: with a dose of pills that are taken once and work for a lifetime. The segment, broadcast on Monday, November 17, 2008, was presented by NBC's chief science and health reporter, Robert Bazell.

"The experiment so far has been only in mice," Bazell reiterated—mice studies are the great bugaboo of medical journalism, because so often the findings cannot be reproduced in humans—"but the results have been exciting. With drugs already on the market to treat cancer, scientists have cured type one diabetes."

Scientists have cured diabetes. Can't you hear the phones ringing at NBC's news studios, from parents who didn't hear the part about mice, calling to get this cure for their kid?

The screen then switched to a close-up of a middle-aged man who looked to be in need of a good night's sleep, with graying hair, a trim gray beard and mustache, and thick, dark eyebrows. "Using drugs that are already approved has the ability potentially to more rapidly move from the benchside [*sic*] to the clinic," said the man, identified as Jeffrey Bluestone, PhD, an immunologist in the Diabetes Center at the University of California, San Francisco. "We didn't have to treat continuously. We could treat for a limited period of time, a couple of months, and then stop the treatment and the animals didn't revert to become diabetic again."

Bazell cautioned again that it was only a preliminary finding, and he introduced a woman, Suzanne Elder, whose young daughter, Sophie, has type 1 diabetes. Bazell said that Elder had heard of cures before, and so she remained skeptical. But Elder said of her daughter, "She has this ongoing, ever-evolving fantasy party we're going to throw for her the day that she's cured. It involves lots of chocolate."

As it happened, I was sitting in Bluestone's office, out of view of the cameras, when the segment was being taped earlier that morning. Bazell did the interview from New York, speaking to Bluestone by speaker phone; only a cameraman and audio engineer showed up for the taping in Bluestone's San Francisco office.

"This is a crazy day because this paper is coming out," Bluestone told me when I arrived at his office around 8:30 A.M. to find the camera crew setting up. "That's a crew from *NBC Nightly News*. Which I find kind of bizarre."

I already knew about the study, from an embargoed press release that had gone out a week earlier, and asked if he thought that having a story about it on a network news show that night was a bit of overkill.

"Whenever it's a mouse, it's overkill," he said. "If it weren't for the fact that we get pressure from the UCSF media people, I wouldn't do it. But I'll underplay it, as you'll see. That's my style."

In fact, if any mouse study merited some hoopla, this one did, as the modest, no-nonsense Bluestone surely knew. Although researchers had previously demonstrated a hundred times over that they could *prevent* type 1 diabetes in mice prone to get it (whether by giving them vitamin D, making their cages messy, or the like), this was only the second time anyone had been able to actually *cure* the disease long-term, with a brief dose of drugs free of toxic complications, whether in mice or any other creature. Truly it was a milestone.

With any other researcher, the discovery might have been written off as just a lucky break, the kind of unexpected, random finding that occasionally falls into a scientist's lap. After all, the effect on diabetes is just a "side effect" of Gleevec, a cancer drug considered so important when approved in 2001 that it was featured on the cover of *Time* magazine. But Bluestone is not just any other researcher. This was only the latest in a series of extraordinary findings that place him squarely on top of the heap of investigators seeking a biological cure of type 1 diabetes and other autoimmune diseases. In fact, another drug, which suppresses an arm of the immune system known as CD3 cells (about which, more later), was actually invented by Bluestone back in the 1980s, and has now been shown to slow the loss of insulin-producing beta cells in humans. Not only in mice, but also in *people.*

As Judith Fradkin, director of diabetes at NIDDK, told me, when asked about the most impressive findings in the field to date, "There have been some home runs, like what Jeff Bluestone did with anti-CD3, where it went from mouse to man. He showed we can actually slow the loss of beta cells in new-onset diabetes. To me, that's really exciting that something moved from mouse to man and actually worked."

100 PERCENT WRONG

Although Bluestone's primary academic appointment is director of UCSF's Diabetes Center, by far his most prestigious, pressure-cooker position is leading a seven-year, $144 million program jointly sponsored by the National Institutes of Health and the Juvenile Diabetes Research Foundation. The Immune Tolerance Network has a truly audacious goal: to not only cure or prevent type 1 diabetes, Crohn's disease, asthma, allergies, and other autoimmune diseases, but to develop drugs and methodologies to permit transplants (including transplants of insulin-producing islet cells) without the need for strong antirejection drugs. Bluestone's mission impossible, in effect, is to master the human immune system.

"If you think about the foundation of the JDRF, it's to cure diabetes and to walk away," Aaron Kowalski, director of research at the JDRF, told me. "Dr. Bluestone was just named a recipient of our Scholars Award, our top award. It's impossible to quantify who is farthest along toward a quote-unquote cure, but he's one of the world's best."

Still, Kowalski pointed out the enormity of the task. "With AIDS and diseases that are viral or bacterial, you're fighting a foreign invader," he said. "The challenge with diabetes is you're fighting yourself. That's where it becomes trickier."

So tricky that some of the top scientific scene-watchers remain skeptical that significant progress can be made toward curing diabetes in anything approaching the short-term. For instance, Richard Kahn, PhD, chief scientific and medical officer of the American Diabetes Association, told me when I visited him at the ADA headquarters outside of Washington, D.C., "I am pessimistic about the ultimate success of preventing autoimmunity, only because I think when you start futzing with the immune system, with our state of knowledge now, it's just going to be really hard to change things and be successful for huge numbers of people. That doesn't mean it's never going to happen. Lots of things we thought never would happen have happened. But it's just tough to find therapies that go deep into cellular methods and not have them result in some serious problems."

Another who expressed skepticism was David Nathan, MD, the Harvard physician-researcher who led the Diabetes Control and Complications Trial. "Fiddling with the immune system—the deeper you go in, the more challenging it seems to be," Nathan said when I visited his office near Massachusetts General Hospital, where he is chief of the diabetes unit. Chewing gum, moving and stretching in his seat, looking every bit the three-times-a-week basketball player he is, Nathan added, "It's a highly evolved—highly, highly, highly, highly complex—system."

Given the skepticism, however, perhaps no one is better suited to take up the challenge of curing diabetes than Bluestone, a researcher whose own radical skepticism toward his and everybody else's theories is legendary and, in scientific circles, greatly admired.

"The reality," he told me, "is I've been proven wrong so many times. Every time I've gone in with a hypothesis on the way I think things work, the biology corrects me. We know so little. We think we know so much. It's just way too presumptuous to think we can predict the answer. Science is about doubt, about questioning the validity of the current state of things. It's something we don't do very well in politics or business, where doubt is always considered a weakness. In science, it's a strength. If we're not willing to question, we're going to miss stuff, because we won't be open to it. I was absolutely sure in the early 'nineties that I knew how to cure diabetes, to block these co-stimulatory pathways that are key to T-cell activation. I was one hundred percent wrong. I remember I got up at a seminar in Harvard, about 1995, and I'll never forget, I said, 'Here's the experiment I did, I absolutely knew what the result would be, and here's the result, it's exactly the opposite. Isn't this great? Now we can figure out what's going on.'"

AN ARMY OF RESEARCHERS

A measure of the task Bluestone has taken on can be found in the experience of Mark Atkinson, PhD, a highly regarded diabetes researcher and professor in the department of pathology, immunology, and laboratory medicine at the University of Florida, Gainesville.

"I'm now twenty-five years into this," Atkinson said. "I know we're a lot closer to a cure than we were, or I was, twenty-five years ago. That said, when I started, people thought we were going to have a cure in a year or two. We had animal models; we were closing in on the genes; we had so many drugs. The disease turned out to be more complex than we thought. There have been a large number of myths about type one diabetes—both treatment myths and cure myths. Alongside of the cure that was coming, the one we still hear so often is when families come in and say, 'My doctor said I got the diabetes virus and that's what caused my disease.' I know old textbooks talk about that, but we don't really know that a virus causes it."

Atkinson, who is currently investigating the use of stem cells drawn from umbilical cord blood, along with half a dozen other strategies, began his career with three goals in mind, he told me. "One was a way to predict who is going to develop diabetes," he said. "Number two was to figure out what causes diabetes; three, find a way to cure or prevent diabetes. I think the field has only found the first one: we now can predict with some certainty who is going to develop diabetes, at least well enough to perform risk studies. The other two—whoa, we're still struggling. I still get emails weekly from parents asking when we'll get a cure." He let loose a sigh. "I get so many emails."

And Atkinson is just one in an army of diabetes researchers across the United States. The JDRF alone spends some $160 million per year on type 1 research, making it the single largest not-for-profit funder of medical research in the world—not just of diabetes research, but of any medical research; by comparison, the American Cancer Society spent 29 percent less, or $124 million, on cancer research and training grants in 2008. What's more, NIDDK, the arm of NIH that funds diabetes research, was budgeted in 2009 at $1.8 billion.

The unofficial headquarters of East Coast diabetes research is surely Boston, home to both the Joslin Diabetes Center and Harvard University. Aside from Nathan, the boldfaced names would have to include a collaborator of his, Denise Faustman, MD, PhD, the lightning-rod director of Mass General's immunology laboratory. As the first to ever claim, back in 2001, the *reversal* of autoimmune diabetes in mice, she met with not only skepticism but outright doubt and derision—the usual soap opera nonsense for which the history of science is famous, dating back to Galileo's condemnation by the Catholic Church for asserting that the earth revolves around the sun. When the JDRF decided not to fund her next big grant proposal, it fell to Lee Iacocca—the former chairman of the Chrysler Corporation, whose wife died of complications from type 1—to convince his foundation to pony up $11.1 million for her proposed study in humans, which she is now running with Nathan.

In 2006, three independent teams published papers confirming Faustman's original claim that after injecting diabetic mice with the treatment she had used—a weakened strain of bacteria that challenges the immune system—many of the mice were cured. In August of 2008, Faustman published an interim paper from her new study in the prestigious *Proceedings of the National Academy of Sciences,* showing that the same treatment worked to stop the autoimmune attack in human cells placed in a test tube. Whether it will ultimately work in living humans remains to be seen, but if Faustman hits one out of the ballpark, many critics will be eating crow, and people with diabetes will be dancing in the streets.

Next on the list of Boston's leading lights in diabetes research would be the field's ultimate power couple, Gordon S. Weir, MD, a Harvard professor who leads both the Diabetes Working Group of the Harvard Stem Cell Institute and Joslin's islet transplantation program, and his wife, Susan Bonner-Weir, PhD, a senior investigator at Joslin and associate professor at Harvard Medical School. In December of 2008, she published a groundbreaking paper in the *Proceedings* showing that duct cells in the pancreas can be prodded to turn into insulin-producing beta cells. Although the study was done in mice, it opens the possibility that within the pancreas of every person with diabetes lurks a reservoir of cells that might one day be induced to turn into beta cells—heady stuff, if confirmed.

Finally, and most famously, there is Douglas A. Melton, MD, co-director of the Harvard Stem Cell Institute, chair of Harvard's department of stem cell and regenerative biology, and twice listed by *Time* magazine among the 100 Most Influential People in the World. Back in 1993, Melton was happily investigating the biology of frog development when his then six-month-old son, Sam, was diagnosed with type 1. Melton responded, daringly, by turning his laboratory upside down to focus on diabetes. His daughter, Emma, was also diagnosed with type 1, in 2001—the same year President George W. Bush announced that no federal funds would support the development of any new lines of human stem cells. Melton promptly found private funds to develop 17 new lines, which he then sent, free of charge, to any laboratory that wanted them. In August of 2008, he reported success in transforming pancreatic cells directly into insulin-producing cells—in mice—and it would be awfully cool if the same trick works in humans.

But there are hundreds of other smart, tenacious, dedicated researchers out there seeking a biological cure of diabetes. Even so, if diabetes research were a sport, Bluestone might well be considered the Michael Jordan of the game.

TREGS AND T CELLS

To spend a day with Bluestone is to witness a scientist in full stride, literally bounding down hallways, fielding media calls, holding video teleconferences, working over scientific manuscripts, touching base with the young scientists in his lab who conduct the many studies he's running, and giving lectures to grad students about the twists and turns of his latest research efforts. By 9:05 A.M. on the day of my visit, Bluestone stood at the podium in his building's ground-floor auditorium, narrating the twists and turns of his latest research efforts for an audience of 100 or so grad students, speaking in a language unintelligible to non-experts.

"To analyze the role of micro RNAs in the development of Tregs," he said at one point, "Xuyu crossed a FoxP3-GFP artificial chromosome transgenic mouse with a Dicer."

Later that morning, after the NBC video crew had packed up and left, Bluestone offered to translate his work into English. We sat in his glass-walled corner office on the 11th floor, a spectacular view of the San Francisco Bay in the background, with a neon sign on the window-sill that said "Club Bluestone" and a signed award on the wall from Mary Tyler Moore (the TV and movie star who was easily the most famous person with type 1 until Nick Jonas of the Jonas Brothers band recently displaced her).

"The immune system," he began, "the adaptive immune system that tackles viruses and bacteria but on occasion induces autoimmunity, is like a big elephant.

"Now we like the immune system when it attacks viruses and bacteria," he continued, "but we don't want it to attack the pancreas. So how are we going to target it? The cluster domains, the CD molecules, are the bull's-eyes on the surface of this particular kind of white blood cell, this elephant. Each cluster domain is a flag that can be attacked by a particular monoclonal antibody. Let's say CD22 is on the foot, CD3 is on the tail, and CD25 is right between the eyes. So we try these different drugs because we think they're going to latch onto these CD molecules and disable the elephant, but we haven't yet fully understood which one is really going to work best. If you hit it right between the eyes and kill the elephant, you know you're going to stop the autoimmune attack on the pancreas. The problem is, if you decapitate the immune system, it can't deal with viruses and bacteria. That's very dangerous. And if you get a drug that just cuts off the tail, it might not do enough to make a real difference. The trick is to find the right CD molecule that, when we disable it, prevents autoimmune disease without killing the whole elephant."

Sweet. And what does that have to do with diabetes? Bluestone tried with another metaphor.

"How did the immune system evolve?" he asked. "It had to have a way to see viruses and bacteria efficiently. What the immune system chose to do was to see very small pieces of those viruses and bacteria, by plucking them down onto this molecule on the surface of every cell in the body, like a hot dog in a bun. It's a very efficient process. The problem is that every time the immune system sees the hot dog—a virus or bacteria—it has to see it in the context of the bun. So it may not be a surprise that at times it makes a mistake and sees the bun too well, which might be in your stomach, or your brain, or your pancreas. So while this system is efficient for seeing bacteria or viruses, it runs the risk of having the immune system see the body itself as foreign."

So the hot dog is the infectious virus or bacteria, the bun is the infected organ, and the mistake occurs when the immune system gets mixed up between the two, and goes on a rampage to destroy the body's own tissue, which, in the case of type 1, is the insulin-producing beta cells in the pancreas.

Luckily, the immune system is made up not only of these vicious attack cells, but also more mild-mannered policing cells that seek to stop unwarranted attacks on the body's own tissue. Bluestone specializes in studying these policing cells, called T regulatory cells, or Tregs. The T stands for thymus, the organ where Tregs are exposed to bits and pieces of every cell in the body, and learn to honor and respect them as "self." Once trained in the thymus, Tregs head off through the bloodstream, looking for any bodily tissues being unfairly set upon by killer T cells, whereupon they release a signal telling the attacking mob to step down. The problem of autoimmunity occurs when Tregs, despite all their training, get lazy, like police officers eating doughnuts when they should be chasing crooks.

That's where Bluestone comes in, seeking to rouse the Tregs from their stupor. He went looking at those cluster domains, or CDs, that sit like targets on the killer T cells. He engineered a monoclonal antibody—a kind of molecular homing pigeon—called teplizumab. Not only does it attack the CD3 receptors on these killer T cells (which is why it's called an "anti-CD3" drug), but it also draws in the Tregs to help them restore the peace.

Bluestone developed teplizumab back in the late 1980s with no thoughts about applying it to diabetes; as a researcher at the University of Chicago, he was simply looking to eliminate the toxic effects of a Johnson & Johnson antirejection drug used in transplants. But in 1994, a French researcher, Lucienne Chatenoud, used Bluestone's drug in NOD mice with autoimmune diabetes and found that it cured their diabetes for months at a time.

"By 1995 we absolutely knew where we wanted to go with it, but J&J shut down the program," Bluestone said. "They had a new head of research who decided—it's funny to think about in retrospect—that monoclonal antibodies were never going to make it commercially. Now the ten best-selling drugs in autoimmune disease are all monoclonal antibodies. It's just crazy. So it went dormant. I had made this stuff myself. It was sitting in the fridge so I was able to keep working on it. But the company wasn't interested."

Finally, in 2004, he was able to buy back the rights to teplizumab, which were then sold to a small biotech company called MacroGenics, which then turned around and sold development rights to Eli Lilly and Company for a neat $44 million up front and as much as $450 million if it gets approved by the FDA and becomes widely used. Meanwhile, during all the years of delay, two other anti-CD3 drugs have also been developed and are now, like teplizumab, in the final stages of testing.

I asked Bluestone if he was bothered by the fact that a drug he invented 20 years ago might now be eclipsed by two copycats.

"It never worries me for a second that there might be another drug that might be better," he said. "It does worry me, though, that we could have had this drug approved ten years ago and been giving it to people. There's no doubt teplizumab slows down the immune attack. In a small percentage of people at the moment there is a really prolonged effect. We have some patients out five years who are still making as much insulin as they made at the beginning. For the most part, though, we see the immune system revving back up after a while. Which is why, in some of the more recent studies, we're focused on giving a second treatment, six months or a year later, to see if giving a second round will prolong the effect in those individuals in whom the drug's effect deteriorates."

Whereas the development of teplizumab was one of rational, intentional design, the story of his latest coup, with the cancer drugs Gleevec and Sutent, was anything but. It began, he said, when he and fellow UCSF researcher Arthur Weiss were sitting out in the parking lot, talking about a friend of Bluestone's who had just been diagnosed with leukemia.

"I was helping her try to decide whether to get a bone marrow transplant or go on this new drug, Gleevec," Bluestone recalled. "She decided to go on Gleevec. A few months later I said, 'Art, she's complaining that her immune system may be screwed up; she has more susceptibility to the common cold.' 'You're an idiot, Jeff,' Art told me. 'We all know it's an immune suppressant. Why aren't you studying this drug in diabetes?' I said, 'Yeah sure.' You never say no to Art.

"We bought some Gleevec. Also bought Sutent, a similar drug. We did the initial experiment in NOD mice, figuring it was a long shot. There are probably 175 different ways to prevent type one in the mouse, but what you really want to do is reverse the disease once they've got it. We saw that in the overwhelming majority, some ninety percent, the disease was reversed in new-onset mice. We stopped the drug, and all these animals became diabetic."

Bluestone went on to describe how he then rolled out the study. "We did a longer treatment group, treated up to ten weeks. When we stopped, a good chunk, a majority, stayed normal glycemic. So how does that work? Being T cell–centric, I thought, of course it affects Tregs. But we couldn't find an effect. Thank God, not everything in my lab is Treg. So what's the target? We don't know the full answer to this."

For all the intellectual work and theory that had led up to the development of teplizumab, in other words, the bottom line was that Bluestone was mystified why Gleevec and Sutent stops the autoimmune attack on insulin-producing beta cells in mice. He just knew it worked.

By 5 P.M. San Francisco time, *NBC Nightly News* had already aired on the East Coast. Bluestone checked his email to see what kind of response it was getting.

"I've already gotten 150 emails," he told me, removing his reading glasses and letting them hang from his neck. "They neglected to say it can only be used in new onset. And it looks like they may have neglected to mention type one versus type two diabetes. So I have to get Jeff Matthews in communications to put something up on our site. It really is a pain in the butt." He rubbed his eyes, looking haggard.

ROAD MAP TO THE FUTURE

Although trained in immunology, Bluestone had little interest in diabetes until the late 1980s, when type 2 started to take a toll on both his mother and father.

"My father started to have many of the complications, and then my mother ended up having a heart attack and dying. That's twenty years ago. She was fifty-three. I had been working on cancer. I thought some of the questions I was asking about cancer, I could be asking in diabetes. And I was also working in organ transplants. I thought, why not do it in islets?"

To this day, he remains close to his father, Jules, who has suffered significant complications from type 2.

"I see him suffering the ravages of the disease. He's lost a leg. He's had eye problems. In 2001, he needed a kidney transplant, which he got from me." That's right: Bluestone donated one of his kidneys to his father. "Now he suffers the ravages of taking the immunosuppressant drugs. He's gotten skin cancers because of them. And then he's had circulation problems from the diabetes. He's lost several digits. He has no feeling in his fingers or legs. It's a pretty bad disease. People who think you just take a little insulin and you're okay don't understand the disease. He just turned eighty. He's still a very active person. He was a life insurance salesman for most of his adult life. Ran a dry-cleaning shop when I was growing up."

In April of 2000, his academic star rising, Bluestone was lured away from the University of Chicago to UCSF with some serious inducements, including private schooling for his two children and jobs at the university for the 12 researchers who worked in his lab.

Married now for 30 years to Leah, a social worker and school counselor, he calls her "the yin to my yang. She's very much a people person, very into sort of the . . . the . . . the touchy-feely stuff, understanding the importance of relationships and people, interfacing. I tend to be a more pragmatic, factual, scientific person with a lot less of the sensitivity of patting people on the back."

Bluestone's tough-nosed attitude applies to his own results as well. Asked point blank whether his anti-CD3 drug, or any of the other anti-CD3 drugs in development, might prove to be a true cure for diabetes, he told me, "There's no doubt the drug is not a magic bullet. I certainly believe that this is not the cure for type one diabetes. It's largely because we're getting in too late. Eighty percent of your islets are destroyed by the time someone is diagnosed with diabetes. There are two things we have to do ultimately. We have to be able to stop the immune attack. Anti-CD3 is pretty good at that. At the same time we have to replace the islets already destroyed, either through a transplant or a drug that increases survival and growth. I also believe in the regeneration area, if we could figure out what the stem cell area is. Susan Bonner-Weir and Gordon Weir are big proponents of duct cells turning into islets. My own feeling is that success will come from being able to take some of the remaining islet cells out, expanding them in vitro, and then injecting them back in."

So what was this High Priest of the effort to find a biological cure for diabetes saying? Will there ever be a cure?

"I truly believe that," he told me. "The road map is there. Every piece has been done at one level or another. I absolutely believe that it's true that we can get cells to turn into insulin-producing cells, we can modify the immune system so it will not attack your pancreas anymore. All those pieces are doable. But whether it's five years or ten years or twenty years, I don't know."

Just before I left his office, shortly after 5:00, with the mid-November sky outside his office window already darkening and the lights on the Golden Gate Bridge coming into view, I asked Bluestone if he saw any larger philosophical implications in his work, as one trying to induce tolerance and peace within the immune system, and why it was so damned difficult.

"If I were religious," he answered, "I might think there is greater work going on here. I do a Google search every day on 'tolerance,' and 'immune tolerance,' to find out what's out there. It's great, because ninety percent of the articles that come back have nothing to do with the immune system, but the Middle East or Southern Baptists or whatever. Tolerance is all over our social fabrics in the world. The reason is the way we and all living things are fundamentally structured to distinguish self from non-self. I don't know what the teleological reason is, although people say it started with sponges, and when they came in touch with each other, for procreation, they had to have a way to distinguish another sponge from other species as foreign."

By June of 2009, just seven months since I'd seen him, Bluestone had published eight more papers in some of the most prominent scientific publications in the world, ranging from the *Proceedings* to *Diabetes, Gut,* and *Clinical Immunology.* None of them had blown the lid off the field, and nothing particularly mind-blowing had come out at the 2009 annual meeting of the American Diabetes Association.

But it's humbling to think that, for all we know, Bluestone or some other researcher just might announce the cure for diabetes in humans tomorrow. As wondrous as that would be, however, any cure will still remain one step short of the ultimate goal of medical research: prevention. Far better to prevent someone from getting cancer, or heart disease, or diabetes in the first place than to treat or cure it afterward. Far better that the children in Weston, Massachusetts, and the

Blankenship family in Logan County, West Virginia, should never have developed diabetes than to cure it after so much worry and suffering. It is to this dream of prevention, of finally reversing the pandemic of type 1 and type 2, that I devote the final chapter of this book.

CHAPTER 13

The Public Health Cure

Prevention Is the Ultimate Key to Ending the Diabetes Pandemic

TO EACH AGE, ITS defining disease. As the Middle Ages had the Black Death, so the 1950s had polio, and the 1980s, AIDS, then wholly untreatable. Back in 1866, when the first urban health agency was formed in the United States, in New York City, the concerns centered around epidemics of cholera, typhoid, smallpox, and tuberculosis, which the Metropolitan Board of Health moved quickly to contain. Today, as the great pandemic of diabetes spreads across the globe, killing more people each day than the H1N1 swine flu pandemic did in its first six months, once again New York is the pioneer.

In February of 2004, a new director arrived at the New York City Department of Health and Mental Hygiene's Bureau of Chronic Disease Prevention and Control with a heretical new mission: to fight diabetes and obesity much as the department had fought smallpox and tuberculosis 100 years earlier: with all the weapons of the public health arsenal.

"The sweet spot in public health is a simple change you can make that is sustainable, practical, and will have a long-term impact," said Lynn A. Silver, MD, who continues to direct the bureau as assistant commissioner of the New York City Department of Health and Mental Hygiene. "A classic example is requiring seat belts. Instead of blaming people for not being good drivers, you make the cars safer. When we started putting together an approach to chronic diseases like diabetes and obesity, our approach was to view them not as individual behavioral issues, but as responses to our environment. We began to ask how we could make sustainable, corrective changes in our environment to help reverse the epidemic."

Silver had grown up in Manhattan but had spent much of her adult life outside the country. Her prior position was as a visiting scholar in the department of international health at the Karolinska Institute, in Stockholm, Sweden. Before that she had lived for 15 years in Brazil, where she worked in public health and had been the dean of a college. It was time now for the local girl to make good in her hometown.

Ideas flew fast and thick in meetings on how to battle diabetes and obesity, but one quickly grabbed Silver's imagination. A proposal had been made in the New York State legislature to require that calorie counts be listed on fast-food menu boards for every item sold. Silver and a colleague, Candace Young wrote a memo in support of the proposal.

The idea, Silver recognized, was simple yet powerful: by prominently displaying how many calories are in each item listed on the menu of a fast-food restaurant, consumers would have better information at the point of sale for making an informed choice. No nagging or finger wagging. Just the facts, ma'am.

She and Young completed the memo for the state legislature in support of their bill. But the state bill didn't go anywhere. Neither did a piece of federal legislation introduced in 2003 by Senator Tom Harkin, Democrat of Iowa, aptly titled the Menu Education and Labeling Act, or MEAL. Predictably, the National Restaurant Association opposed Harkin's bill, and it died with hardly a whisper of news coverage.

But Silver was hooked on the idea, and she began to investigate whether New York City's health department could mandate calorie counts posted on fast-food menu boards *without* any new legislation. "It was clear we had this long-standing authority to assure food safety in the restaurant sector," she said. "It had traditionally been used for infectious disease prevention. But we argued that we could use this same, existing authority for chronic disease prevention."

Some in the department weren't so sure. Setting sanitary requirements is one thing, but where was it written that the city could force restaurants to place calorie information on their menu boards?

"A hundred and fifty years ago," Silver told me, "when tuberculosis was rampant in New York City, new rules were written for housing and sanitation. That was part of the origins of modern public health. It was very difficult and a big change at the time, but it was needed to address the health problems of the day. I didn't think we should be afraid of reconceiving what our environmental challenges are today, which include our food environment."

After two years of research, meetings, and debate, a consensus was reached in Silver's department that this was an issue they could and should get behind. There was just one problem. First, they would have to convince Wilfredo Lopez, the department's longtime, white-haired general counsel, that the action was not only a good thing for the public health, but wouldn't get them laughed out of court in the highly likely event that the fast-food corporations dragged them there.

BLAMING THE VICTIM

"If you have a problem like diabetes, it's your own fault."

Kelly D. Brownell, PhD, was giving voice to the powerful and pervasive view, usually spoken only behind people's backs, that for decades has been the secret fuel behind self-help books, medical care, and countless family feuds over why Grandpa, or Mom, or even little Joey has type 2 diabetes. Typically, of course, the view is couched in its more politely positive corollary: that if you dug yourself into that hole, by golly, you can dig yourself out with a little willpower and a nifty new diet. Brownell, however, has devoted his career—he is now professor of psychology, epidemiology, and public health at Yale, and director of its Rudd Center for Food Policy and Obesity—to elucidating why the personal-responsibility approach, however alluring it may be, simply falls a few notches short on the belt buckle.

"It's like telling people who live near a factory that's spewing out pollutants not to breathe the air," he told me. "Sure, in any public health matter, you have to rely on people's discipline, restraint, and willpower to some extent. But you get to the point where you realize that's not enough. You have to affect the environmental conditions that are driving the behavior."

As if anyone needs convincing that it is hard to permanently change eating habits because of what a doctor, a nagging spouse, or a bathroom scale might say, a recent study in the *Archives of Internal Medicine* showed how hard it is. While almost one in three smokers quit cigarettes following a stroke or the diagnosis of cancer, heart disease, or lung disease, the study found, obese or overweight people managed to lose only two or three pounds on average after being diagnosed with diabetes or heart disease. *It's harder to quit overeating, apparently, than to quit smoking.*

Why is that? Although we often assume the battle of the bulge to be a fair fight between us and that ice-cream cone, in fact, there are unseen agents in the cone's corner. In addition to the hormonal influences arising from the intestines, as described in chapter 11, there are also potent psychological influences manipulated by food marketers who have carefully researched every trick in the book for making you "choose" to buy that cone instead of, say, raspberries. Of your own free will.

"Most of us are blissfully unaware of what influences how much we eat," writes Brian Wansink, PhD, in his eye-opening and hilarious book *Mindless Eating: Why We Eat More Than We Think*. As director of the Cornell University Food and Brand Lab, Wansink has conducted dozens of devilishly clever studies showing how easily we are manipulated by what he calls the "hidden influencers." As he writes, "We all think we're too smart to be influenced by packages, lighting, or plates . . . . We are almost never aware that it is happening to us."

My favorite of Wansink's many studies was published in October 2007 in the *Journal of Consumer Research*. He and Pierre Chandon, a French researcher, asked people to estimate how many calories were in a sandwich from Subway, famous for making health claims in its advertisements, compared to a sandwich from McDonald's. They estimated that the Subway sandwich had 35 percent fewer calories than the one from McDonald's—but in reality, the two items contained nearly the same amount of calories. What's more, Wansink found, they ordered side dishes containing more than *twice* as many calories from the supposedly "healthy" Subway than from the "unhealthy" McDonald's.

So our guts are against us, our minds are against us, and the food companies are against us. Have we left anyone out? Oh yeah. Our friends and families are against us too. A recent study in the *New England Journal of Medicine* found that over the course of 32 years, a person's chance of becoming obese jumps by 57 percent if he or she has a friend who becomes obese, 40 percent if a sibling becomes obese (no matter how far away that sibling lives), and 37 percent if a spouse does. Neighbors had little influence; friends and family members of the same sex had more influence than those of the opposite sex; and statistically significant effects could be seen even from friends-of-friends.

Of course, the same study also found that friends and families who *lost* weight imparted a similarly powerful influence on people's odds of losing weight themselves. Either way, though, the implication is the same: we're all in this together.

PERSUADING MR. LOPEZ

Given the power of these invisible influencers, it should not be surprising that Lynn Silver thought it might be helpful to bring some of them, such as calorie information, out in the open. By no means was she alone in liking the idea. Without the support of New York's mayor, Michael Bloomberg, such an innovative step would have been a nonstarter. And the health commissioner, Thomas R. Frieden, MD, MPH, had likewise made a name for himself as a staunch advocate of public health measures since joining the department as an assistant commissioner in 1992, when he implemented tough new rules to control the city's then-burgeoning tuberculosis epidemic. Soon after being promoted to lead the department, in 2002, he made national headlines by spearheading efforts to ban smoking in almost all public places. And in 2006, under his leadership, the city's Board of Health voted to ban trans fats from all foods served in restaurants, the first city in the nation to do so. It was Frieden, after all, who established the department's Bureau of Chronic Disease Prevention and Control, and who tasked Silver with proposing innovative new strategies to fight diabetes and obesity.

Another strong supporter of Silver's plan to require calorie counts on menu boards was Mary Bassett, MD, MPH, deputy commissioner for Health Promotion and Disease Prevention. "The whole last century in public health represented a shift in emphasis from communicable diseases to chronic diseases," Bassett told me. "Just as people have thought for decades that government should take a role in assuring that the air we breathe is healthful, the water we drink is healthful, people are increasingly seeing a government role for assuring that the food we eat is healthy in its nutritional content. It's a return to public health picking up old tools of environmental interventions that were used so successfully to tackle the communicable disease burden."

The one sticking point in the department, it turned out, was Mr. Lopez, the general counsel. He had no problem with the motive behind such a move, but he was concerned about the legality of requiring it. "Sure, the underlying health rationale was undeniable," he told me. "Super-sizing and all that was having a deleterious health impact on New Yorkers." But, he said, "My first reaction was why pick on fast-food restaurants? I was thinking that if they were to challenge the provision, they would say it's selective prosecution, that there's no basis for limiting it just to fast-food restaurants."

Having joined the health department in 1979 as a staff attorney and worked his way up to general counsel by 1992, Lopez had seen firsthand how messy these matters could get once they reached the courtroom. It wasn't that he disliked the idea of requiring calories to be posted on menu boards; he just wasn't sure it was *legally defensible.*

"Most people think the role of lawyers is to gum up the works," he said. "I tried to be helpful when I could."

Back in the 1980s, when the department was considering banning smoking in restaurants, the idea was floated to limit the ban to larger establishments with seating for 35 patrons or more.

"When we looked at that proposal, we said, you know, it would make more sense for a legislature to enact that," Lopez said, "because that's not so much a health-based distinction, between smaller and larger restaurants, as an economic distinction. So we went to the city council and got a local law enacted." The wisdom of seeking a new law was demonstrated soon after, when the state board of health tried to enforce a similar ban without one; the New York State legislature actually fought the move in court and had the rules outside of New York City overturned.

"So I was sensitive to making sure that if we apply new rules to only fast-food restaurants," he said, "these kinds of distinctions not be based on strictly economic grounds." If the department attempted to exempt mom-and-pop restaurants from listing calorie counts on their menus simply on the grounds that it would pose an undue economic burden on them, Lopez knew, it would get thrown out in court. The department of health's powers extended only over matters of *health,* not *economics.*

And so the idea remained in limbo, stalled on Lopez's desk, until one evening when a farewell party was held for a departing colleague in the department and the health commissioner, Thomas Frieden, said something that caused a "Eureka" moment for Lopez.

"Dr. Frieden usually stops in for about half an hour at those things and then goes back to the office," Lopez told me. "But I recall we were at this function and he again raised the topic. He is not one to let a good idea blithely ride off into the sunset. He said to me, 'But you know, Wilfredo, the fast-food restaurants are the only ones for which it makes sense, because there the portions and the content are standardized.' To me, that was like a light bulb going on. That created a rational basis for the distinction. In fact, fast-food restaurants were the only places for which the posting of calories was operationally feasible."

It wasn't just that the menus at the large fast-food chains are *consistent*, he realized, but that the food items themselves are *virtually identical*, no matter where they are purchased. "A Quarter Pounder with cheese is the same size and has the same ingredients at one McDonald's as another," Lopez said. "Whereas in a mom-and-pop restaurant, you might have somebody trying to cut the steak in equal sizes, but they're really not consistent enough."

That realization armed him with the defensible legal basis he needed, so Lopez and New York City's health department publicly proposed its plan in September of 2006 to establish the first rule in the United States requiring fast-food restaurants to list calories on their menu boards. A few months later, on Tuesday, December 5, the city's Board of Health voted to approve it. That Friday, as it happened, was Lopez's last day on the job; after more than 25 years, he had decided to retire. Six months later, when the New York State Restaurant Association filed suit to block the action, he would have to watch from the sidelines to see whether the final craftwork of his legal career would stand up in court.

REGULATING FAST FOOD LIKE POLLUTION

Menu boards are hardly the only place where public health advocates are hitting the fast-food restaurants. A more direct, but more difficult, strategy seeks to limit the sheer number of outlets. In a place like Logan County, with the highest rate of diabetes in the country, the 36 fast-food restaurants, serving a population of less than 38,000, stand out like foreign forts of an occupying army, their sparkling, fresh appearance strikingly at odds with the dismal, down-and-out look of many homes and local businesses.

When clustered to the exclusion of more wholesome food outlets, the unhealthful impact of these chains—and yes, the double meaning is intended—can be surprisingly strong. A Canadian study published in June of 2009, for instance, found that as the ratio of fast-food restaurants and convenience stores goes up in comparison to supermarkets and specialty food stores (where more healthful foods can be purchased), the risk of obesity of people living nearby also goes up. The effect, however, was quite local, holding strongly within a half-mile radius of a person's home, but not beyond that boundary.

Another study, presented at a recent meeting of the American Stroke Association, found that the risk of stroke increases with the number of fast-food restaurants in a neighborhood. Even after controlling for all the predictable economic and social factors, the study found that in neighborhoods with the highest number of fast-food restaurants, residents had a 13 percent higher risk of suffering a stroke than those living in areas with the lowest numbers of the chains.

To fight such influences, lawmakers around the country have proposed a variety of measures, some of them frankly harebrained. In Mississippi, for instance, State Representative John Read, a Republican, co-sponsored a bill in 2008 that would have banned restaurants from serving food to obese individuals. "I was trying to shed a little light on the No. 1 problem in Mississippi," Read said, noting that the state has the highest obesity rate in the nation. In the uproar that immediately followed, the chairman of the state's House Public Health and Human Services Committee pronounced the bill "dead on arrival at my desk."

Better thinking went into a bill proposed to place a one-year moratorium on the opening of any new fast-food restaurants in

South Los Angeles. The bill was put forward by city councilwoman Jan Perry, who told the *Washington Post*, "Some people will say, 'Well, people just don't have to eat it.' But the fact of the matter is, what if you have no other choices?" She cited evidence showing that 45 percent of restaurants in the South L.A. area were fast-food outlets, compared to 16 percent in upscale West L.A. In July of 2008, the council approved the one-year moratorium, with extensions possible that could keep the ban in place for an additional year.

Another tactic being eyed by advocates, as yet without success, is restricting television commercials for fast foods or junk foods, particularly those aimed at children or aired during children's programming. A careful analysis published in the *Journal of Law and Economics* in November of 2008 concluded that a total ban on all TV commercials for fast-food restaurants would cut the prevalence of overweight among children between the ages of three and 11 by 18 percent, and among adolescents by 14 percent. Because the cost of such advertising is currently tax deductible as a business expense, the study analyzed what would happen if the IRS simply stopped allowing such a deduction. Assuming the companies continued to spend the same amount on commercials, they would be forced to air fewer commercials; the reduction, the study concluded, would still result in 5 percent to 7 percent fewer children being overweight.

Banning Ronald McDonald from the airways, however, would be a cinch compared to the bigger struggle, the mother of all food fights, being advocated by leaders of the movement for healthier food policies, among them Kelly Brownell, Marion Nestle (the New York University professor and author of *Food Politics* and *What to Eat*), Alice Waters (chef, co-owner of Chez Panisse, and longtime proponent of natural and locally grown foods), and Michael Pollan (a neighbor of Waters's in Berkeley, where he is a professor of journalism and best-selling author of, most recently, *In Defense of Food: An Eater's Manifesto*).

Separately and together, these healthy-food proponents have been outspoken critics of federal farm subsidies that support giant grain and corn farmers. The subsidies not only make for cheaper bread, but for cheaper chips, high-fructose corn sweetener, and grain-fed cattle—all at the expense, they point out, of healthier fruits and vegetables. As a result of such policies, Brownell told me, "An entree salad costs more than a Big Mac value meal. The fundamental economics of food is tipped on its head. If the salad cost half the price of the Big Mac meal, you know a lot more people would be eating salad."

Professor Nestle, in particular, has taken aim at ineffectual government health programs that spew recommendations for *what people should eat,* rather than setting standards for *what food companies can market.* "Advice focused on individuals has not succeeded in reversing current health trends," she wrote in the *American Journal of Public Health,* in an editorial entitled "Preventing Childhood Diabetes: The Need for Public Health Intervention." The time has come, she argued, for government regulators to take on the food companies directly.

WINNING A BATTLE

After all the work of Wilfredo Lopez, Lynn Silver, and others in New York City's health department to craft the rule requiring calories to be posted on fast-food menu boards, the restaurant association filed suit against the measure in June of 2007. A ruling in favor of the restaurant association came just three months later, from Judge Richard J. Holwell of Federal District Court in Manhattan. The problem, it turned out, was that the city had tried to be *too* considerate, demanding only that chains that had previously listed calorie contents of menu items on their brochures, tray liners, posters, or websites would now have to do so on their menu boards. The restaurant association had argued—and Judge Holwell agreed—that voluntary disclosure of calorie information fell under the guidelines of a federal law: the Nutrition Labeling and Education Act of 1990. While the NLEA placed firm requirements on how makers of prepared foods sold in supermarkets must present their nutritional information, it expressly allowed restaurants wide discretion in how to present the information—if they chose to present it at all.

Even so, Judge Holwell virtually invited the city to rejigger its regulation in a way that would move it out from under the penumbra of the NLEA. Instead of basing its requirement on whether or not restaurants had previously made a *voluntary* disclosure, the city could impose "a blanket mandatory duty on all restaurants meeting a standard definition such as operating 10 or more restaurants under the same name," he wrote. In response, Health Commissioner Frieden quipped to the *Times,* "You could say with the judge's ruling we lost this battle, but it became more likely that we would win the war."

And so it was: in April of 2008, Judge Holwell ruled in favor of the Board of Health's new plan to require calories posted on menu boards of all restaurants with at least 15 outlets nationwide. Even with Judge Holwell's decision, however, questions remained about the ultimate fate of the menu labeling law. True, New York City health inspectors soon went about handing out violation notices—to a Dunkin' Donuts at 445 Park Avenue South, a Popeye's at 321 West 125th Street, a Sbarro next to the Empire State Building, and two other outlets. But the restaurant association wasn't ready to give up the fight. The group filed an appeal to a federal appellate court, and legal pundits set to handicapping the odds that they might yet prevail. The final ruling would not come for nearly a year.

WAR ON INACTIVITY

Preventing type 2 diabetes is not just about food, of course. There are the other issues, such as ensuring adequate levels of vitamin D and limiting exposure to persistent organic pollutants, addressed in Part 2 of this book. The other biggie is *energy expenditure:* figuring out ways to get people to burn more of the calories they so efficiently consume.

Way back in 1980, Kelly Brownell of Yale's obesity center undertook a study which, at the time, no other researcher had ever attempted:

seeing if he could convince ordinary people to take the stairs instead of an escalator at public buildings with just one dumb sign. He undertook the study in Philadelphia, in a commuter train station, a bus terminal, and a city shopping mall called the Gallery.

"At each of these places, stairs and escalators were side by side," he told me. "We wanted to think of a message that could be communicated quickly, to encourage people to use the stairs."

After much puzzling over the matter, he decided to contact Tony Auth, the Pulitzer prize–winning editorial cartoonist for the Philadelphia *Inquirer*. In all of about ten minutes, Auth came up with an adorable sketch of two little guys who looked like cartoon hearts. One of them was tired and overweight, slouching on an escalator; the other was buff and smiling, running up an escalator. "YOUR HEART NEEDS EXERCISE," the caption said. "HERE'S YOUR CHANCE."

With the agreement of authorities, Dr. Brownell and his colleagues proceeded to watch people use the stairs or escalators before the poster was put in place, and again while it was up. In all, they made 45,694 observations of people using either the stairs or an adjacent escalator. With the simple addition of Auth's poster, they found, "We just about *tripled* the number of people who would use the stairs."

Although Brownell never followed up on the results, dozens of other researchers did. One of the most prolific in the field has been Frank Eves, PhD, senior lecturer in applied psychology at the School of Sport and Exercise Sciences at the University of Birmingham, England. Since being asked by the World Health Organization in 1997 to review the science of how best to encourage people to engage in more physical activity, he has taken up the subject and, er, run with it.

"At that time there wasn't very much good evidence from randomized trials," Professor Eves told me. "The Brownell study was the original. That's what got me interested, that it looked like such a simple intervention that actually works."

At this point, Eves knows of at least 26 studies in which researchers attempted a simple intervention—usually nothing more than a sign or a banner—to get people in public buildings to use stairs rather than an escalator. "It turns out that at last count, twenty-four of twenty-six studies show it works unequivocally," he said. However, he was quick to point out, only a handful of studies have been done on the tougher challenge: getting people to use stairs instead of an elevator (or, as he called it, a "lift"). "There's no doubt in my mind you can get people with signage to take the stairs rather than the lift at work," he said. "So far, though, we have two studies published and one almost in press."

The beauty of the approach, he said, is that few people think of stair climbing as exercise. "People don't realize just how intense it is as exercise," he said. "We've argued that people mindlessly will choose the escalator or the lift. By changing the context at the point of choice with a brightly colored sign, we can interrupt this mindless behavior."

I asked him whether he thought managers of office buildings, hotels, malls, and other public spaces should try putting up posters near the elevators to encourage people to take the stairs.

"To change people's behavior is not that easy," he said. "It depends on what the message is, and whether it's seen as a top-down message from the management to get people to take the stairs. People never like that. You can't tell people what to do; you can only point out what they might do. You can't preach to people and make them do it. It has to be their choice."

In New York City, a similar effort to get people moving can be seen on many of Manhattan's broad avenues, where specially designated bike lanes have taken over street space once allocated to automobiles. And in newly designed suburbs, a movement is afoot to place side-walks on every street and to locate stores and schools centrally, in order to encourage more walking.

Another front in the war on inactivity is the school gymnasium, where children have been spending precious little time in recent years (unless one counts the use of gyms for lunchrooms). Public health groups recommend that elementary school students have at least 30 minutes of physical education *every day,* and that middle and high school students get at least 45 minutes a day. But according to the CDC's 2006 School Health Policies and Programs Study, fewer than 4 percent of elementary school students, 8 percent of middle school students, and a hair over 2 percent of high school students spend that much time in phys ed. As an outstanding article by Associated Press reporter Nancy Armour revealed in June of 2009, only two states, Illinois and Massachusetts, currently require all schoolchildren to attend at least some physical education. "Some educators complain that physical education—along with art and music—has been squeezed out by No Child Left Behind," Armour wrote.

Perhaps the law's unintended consequence, it occurred to me, was to leave no child behind in the United States' great march toward obesity and diabetes.

JUDGMENT DAY

By mid-2009, the menu labeling rules that Lynn Silver, of New York City's health department, had championed were already demonstrating clear benefits to New Yorkers. In the spring of 2008, before the rules took effect, only 23 percent of consumers surveyed by the health department said that they had seen calorie information inside a Subway, Starbucks, or 15 other chains. After the regulation went into effect, that number jumped to 60 percent. The largest increase was at burger chains, where only 30 percent said they saw calorie information before the rules went into effect, compared to 76 percent after.

Better yet, about one-fourth of those who saw the information after the rule took effect said *it affected what they bought,* which the health department estimated would translate into about 139,000 more people seeing and using the information each day than would have prior to the regulation.

Moreover, the efforts of the Big Apple to push back against the Big Mac have had national repercussions. The state of California has now passed a similar law requiring chain restaurants to post calories on their menus, as have a growing list of localities, including Seattle; Portland, Oregon; and Westchester County, New York. And although the National Restaurant Association opposed each of those bills, it has now gotten behind the 2009 version of Senator Harkin's MEAL bill, primarily because the federal law would supersede all local bills, including New York City's.

Dr. Silver told me she didn't mind that the rule she had worked so hard to put in place in New York might soon be relegated to history because "the final negotiated version of the federal bill doesn't look too bad." Indeed, she added, "It's been very gratifying to be able to propose a policy change, to work in an environment that's been so supportive of that kind of innovative thinking, and to see it come to fruition. There are outbreaks like swine flu we don't like, and outbreaks of menu board posting that we do like."

Federal legislation was also under consideration during the summer of 2009 to impose a new tax on soda and other sweetened drinks as part of what the Senate Finance Committee called "lifestyle tax proposals." Not only the soft-drink lobby was working hard against the bill, but also the corn-refiners' lobby, because high-fructose corn syrup is used in making soda.

Meanwhile, New York State Health Commissioner Richard Daines became an unlikely YouTube sensation with a video (easily found by just typing Daines's name into Google or YouTube), in which he talks about the dangers of sweetened soda with some funny props and bargain-basement production values. Pulling out cans of soda, glasses of milk, and a brownish blob of rubbery fat, he explains how the typical New Yorker's increased intake of just three additional cans per week of sweetened soda results in an additional 21,000 calories per year, which becomes, he says, "about six pounds of fat—and that's just one year's worth." Shaking the squiggly blob of fat, he says, "Good luck trying to hide this on an adult, let alone a child."

As Professor Brownell sees it, "There is tremendous momentum at the moment. A number of factors have converged." Besides the growing awareness that public policy–makers can and must take action to fight the rising rates of obesity and diabetes, Brownell pointed to President Obama's decision to appoint Thomas Frieden, New York's health commissioner, in charge of the Centers for Disease Control and Prevention. Together, the many efforts give him hope that a new trend is underway.

"If you think of this as a line or curve," he told me, "it hits a critical mass and escalates really rapidly. That's what we hope for and expect."

An important new step came on July 28, 2009, when Health and Human Services Secretary Kathleen Sebelius announced that "significant" federal funds will be committed to fighting obesity. As part of the Obama administration's economic stimulus plan, she said, the better part of $1 billion will be funneled to a CDC effort to fighting obesity, heart disease, and other chronic conditions.

And what about that appeal the New York State Restaurant Association filed against the menu posting rule? On Tuesday, February 17, 2009, a federal appellate court rejected it, removing the last shadow of uncertainty that had hung over the rule. Although little was made of it at the time, the makeup of the appellate panel was rather unusual. The Second Circuit had designated that it would be made up of Judge Rosemary S. Pooler, who wrote the decision; Chief Judge Jane A. Restani of the United States Court of International Trade; and another judge from the Second Circuit: Sonia Sotomayor. Just over three months later, Judge Sotomayor was nominated by President Obama for appointment to the U.S. Supreme Court, which made for a bit of history: she would be the first Justice on the nation's highest bench to have type 1 diabetes.

CONCLUSION

I N CLOSING, LET'S TAKE a brief look back at where we began: with 10 children who developed type 1 diabetes in 24 months within two miles of one another in the upscale suburbs of Boston. Rather than bemoan their fate, parents there organized and asked for an investigation to be conducted by the state, which is ongoing. Among those who have participated in organizing meetings are Ray Allen, the Celtics star, and his wife, Shannon, whose son, Walker, was the seventh child diagnosed there.

"Shannon and Ray have turned out to be the most incredible advocates," Ann Marie Kreft recently told me. "We have fabulous people on board who are spending inordinate amounts of their time on advocacy."

I asked her what they are advocating for. "I think we all agree that mandatory case reporting would be the ideal," she said. "That would be the dream come true. I think we may be building up to that."

Rather than have to design a special survey every time an apparent cluster of type 1 cases emerges, mandatory case reporting, on a national level, would permit the CDC to automatically track cases as they emerge, to see not only the big national picture, but also local variations that could prove crucial in unraveling the riddle of why type 1 diabetes continues to rise, each and every year, by 3 percent.

Presently, however, no national organization is advocating for mandated case reporting of type 1. Where is the line of protesters holding placards, marching outside the Atlanta offices of the CDC?

Perhaps we need to look farther back, to the period before the diabetes pandemic began. In 1866, you might recall, the death rate from diabetes in New York City was 1.3 per 100,000 residents. If that rate held today for the 306 million residents of the United States, there would be 4,284 deaths due to diabetes each year. Instead, in 2006, there were 72,507 death certificates on which diabetes was listed as the underlying cause. The official national death rate from diabetes now stands at 23.3 per 100,000, according to the CDC—nearly 19 times higher than it was following the Civil War. And that doesn't count the additional 200,000 or so deaths each year for which diabetes is listed as a "contributing" cause.

Why are none of America's 23 million people with diabetes demanding a federal investigation of this ongoing rise? Has the time not come to recognize that we are all in this together, and that we need to speak up and demand, as Jeffrey Brewer did when he went to meetings of academics studying the artificial pancreas, that researchers and federal officials stop the dithering?

Much as I understand the FDA's need to establish the safety and effectiveness of any new device, I must say that I find it incomprehensible, ridiculous, and simply outrageous that an automatic shut-off for insulin pumps, when sugar levels are falling dangerously low, isn't already available in the United States today. This is the kind of business-as-usual delay that people with AIDS stopped putting up with from federal health officials years ago.

While the American Diabetes Association can and does support public health campaigns and legislation, the focus of its monthly magazine, like the focus of virtually all medical efforts to improve the lot of people with diabetes, is self-management. Here's a new meter; now test your sugars. Here's a new recipe; now count your carbs. And who can argue with the view that people must take control of their diabetes? No one. It's a given that people with diabetes must be their own primary caregiver.

But it's just as clear—or at least I hope it is by now—that focusing on personal responsibility alone has not stopped, and will never stop, the rise of diabetes. *Something more is needed:* recognition that forces beyond the individual's control are at play, and that united action is necessary to face down what is a public, and therefore political, danger to our well-being, and to the well-being of our children.

"People with issues like diabetes can be very powerful agents of their own change but also of national change," Yale's Professor Brownell told me. "Unfortunately that power often gets exercised through professional organizations like the ADA. People with these problems can take part in advocacy movements, even form their own groups to say, 'We don't want junk-food product placement in movies, we don't want our kids going to junk-food websites, we want access to healthy foods that are affordable.' Sometimes these advocacy groups, like Mothers Against Drunk Driving, can have a very powerful political voice."

And so I offer up this name for a new kind of organization: Citizens United in Resolve to End Diabetes.

ACKNOWLEDGMENTS

T HIS BOOK COULD NOT have been written without the participation of hundreds of physicians, researchers, parents, and people with diabetes who kindly gave me their time, welcoming me into their homes or offices to share their insights, experiences, and expertise. To all those named and unnamed in the book, I extend my thanks.

In particular, I wish to thank the families and patients in the suburbs of Boston, including Weston and Woburn, who have struggled with the cluster of type 1 cases there (especially Ann Marie Kreft, who facilitated many of my meetings and interviews); and the gracious people of Logan, West Virginia (especially the Blankenships).

At the library of the New York Academy of Medicine, Miriam Mandelbaum, curator of Rare Books and Manuscripts, was of great help in finding original documents related to the history of diabetes.

At the American Diabetes Association, Diane Tuncer facilitated interviews with senior scientific officers, and gave me full access to back issues of the organization's consumer magazine, *Diabetes Forecast.*

At the Joslin Diabetes Center in Boston, enlightening interviews with Martin J. Abrahamson, Lori Laffel, Rohit Kulkarni, Enrique Caballero, and Donald M. Barnett were arranged by Kira Jastive. Rachel Joslin Whitehouse, who also works at the center and is Dr. Elliott Joslin's great-granddaughter, gave me a great tour.

At the Juvenile Diabetes Research Foundation, Aaron Kowalski was of enormous help, not only in answering all my many questions, but in facilitating interviews with others involved in the JDRF's Artificial Pancreas Project.

At the Banting House National Historic Site of Canada in London, Ontario, curator Grant M. Maltman gave me an inspiring and informative tour.

Leading researchers at both the National Institute of Diabetes Digestive and Kidney Diseases and the Centers for Disease Control and Prevention were astonishingly generous with their time, answering every question I put to them.

Danielle Sudan shared the story of how her 16-year-old brother, Thomas, tragically died in the hospital on the very day he was diagnosed with type 2 diabetes. Dr. Brad Harris shared the devastating story of trying to save a young girl from the same fate.

Two fellow journalists with type 1 diabetes, Miriam E. Tucker and James S. Hirsch (author of the excellent book *Cheating Destiny*), allowed me to pick their brains and gave me great feedback. It was Jim who first told me about the cluster of type 1 cases in Weston.

Two friends and neighbors who also have type 1 diabetes, Michael Mernin and Barbara Werner, have been great comrades in arms against this stupid disease.

Kelly Close of Close Concerns shared her perspective not only as a person with type 1, but as a publisher, editor, and writer of newsletters about the disease. I heartily recommend her patient-oriented electronic newsletter, diaTribe, at *www.diatribe.us*.

Celia Vimont, Mike Hurley, and Maureen Sgambati were early readers of the manuscript and gave invaluable advice.

Thanks to Matthew Lore for first suggesting to me the idea of writing a work of narrative, investigative journalism about the diabetes pandemic.

Thanks as always to my terrific agent, Jane Dystel, for her tenacity and faith in me. Thanks, also, to Don Fehr, editorial director of Kaplan Publishing, for his vision and support, and to all the talented folks at Kaplan who have brought this book to fruition.

To Dr. Zachary Bloomgarden, clinician and medical editor par excellence, who wrote the foreword to this book, and who has been my physician for going on 25 years: thanks for your extraordinary care and knowledge. Dr. Bloomgarden's longtime staff, Vera and Roxanne, are just the best.

To my father-in-law, John Garbarini, who worked for many years as a chemist, developing antibiotics and other life-saving drugs: I always enjoy our discussions about science, especially when they devolve into arguments.

To my wife, Alice, and our lovely and talented daughter, Annie: thank you for your love and encouragement, and I look forward to spending a lot more time with you both now that this book is finished.

Finally, I wish to thank the one who has stayed by my side throughout the research and writing process, literally sitting at my feet: our dog, whose name, of course, is Sugar.

ENDNOTES

FOREWORD

Page

x   *Kelly West, who many consider...* Kelly McGuffin West, *Epidemiology of Diabetes and Its Vascular Lesions* (New York: Elsevier, 1978).

PROLOGUE

Page

xiii   *Twelve miles west of Boston lies its wealthiest suburb...* www.massbenchmarks. org/statedata/data/median99.pdf. (Accessed on July 19, 2009.)

xiii   *13 soccer fields...* www.westonsoccer.org/. (Accessed on August 1, 2009.)

xiii   *19 baseball diamonds...* www.eteamz.com/westonbaseball/locations/. (Accessed on August 1, 2009.)

xiii   *the state's best public school system...* Katherine Ozment, "The Best High Schools," *Boston Magazine,* September 2004, *www.bostonmagazine.com/ articles/public_vs_private_the_best_high_schools/.* (Accessed on August 1, 2009.)

xiii   *nearly 500 classes a year...* http://weston.govoffice.com/. (Accessed on August 1, 2009.)

xiii   *Rikki Conley...* The narrative and quotations from Rikki Conley, Ann Marie Kreft, and others in Weston and its surrounding suburbs are based on numerous interviews I conducted in person and via email and telephone.

xvi   *for every 100,000 children in a given area, about 19 new cases...* Centers for Disease Control and Prevention: National Diabetes Fact Sheet, 2007, *www .cdc.gov/diabetes/pubs/pdf/ndfs_2007.pdf.* (Accessed on July 19, 2009.)

xvii   *an open letter of support to Ray Allen...* James S. Hirsch, "Living, Growing, and Learning to Live with Diabetes," *Boston Globe,* July 7, 2008.

xvii   *Ann Marie and her husband published a letter...* Ann Marie Kreft, Tim Ramsey, and Kathy Richard, "Diabetes Registry, More Research Can Help Ailing Children," *Boston Globe,* July 17, 2008.

xviii   *the infamous lawsuit featured in the book and movie...* Jonathan Harr, *A Civil Action* (New York: Random House, 1995).

xviii   *Erin Brockovich vigor...* Gretchen Voss, "Outbreak," *Boston Magazine,* February 2009, *www.bostonmagazine.com/articles/outbreak/page2.* (Accessed on Aug. 4, 2009.)

xx   *Type 1... about twice as common...* These estimates are based on interviews with dozens of leading researchers, many of whom are quoted elsewhere in the book, and a review of dozens of studies, including Edwin A. M. Gale, "The Rise of Childhood Type 1 Diabetes in the 20th Century," *Diabetes* 51 (December 2002): 3353–61; Ronny A. Bell, Elizabeth J. Mayer-Davis, Jennifer W. Beyer, et al., "Prevalence, Incidence, and Clinical Characteristics: The SEARCH for Diabetes in Youth Study," *Diabetes Care* 32, Supplement (2009): S102–S111; Kendra Vehik, Richard F. Hamman, MD, Dennis Lezotte, et al., "Increasing Incidence of Type 1 Diabetes in 0- to 17-Year-Old Colorado Youth," *Diabetes Care* 30 (2007): 503–509.

xx   *CDC now projects that 33 percent of all boys...* K. M. Venkat Narayan, James P. Boyle, PhD, and Theodore J. Thompson, "Lifetime Risk for Diabetes Mellitus in the United States," *Journal of the American Medical Association* 290, no. 4 (2003): 1884–90.

xx   *At Children's Hospital in Cincinnati...* O. Pinhas-Hamiel, L. M. Dolan, S. R. Daniels, et al., "Increased Incidence of Non-Insulin-Dependent Diabetes Mellitus Among Adolescents," *Journal of Pediatrics* 128 (May 1996): 608–15.

xx   *the percent of adolescent girls receiving prescription medications for type 2...* Miranda Hitti, "Prescription Drug Use Up in Teen Girls," CBS News, May 17, 2007, *www.cbsnews.com/stories/2007/05/17/health/webmd/main2823481.shtml.* (Accessed on July 19, 2009.)

xx   *Reports of kids dying due to diabetes...* See, for instance, Rebecca M. Carchman, Martha Dechert-Zeger, Ali S. Calikoglu, et al., "A New Challenge in Pediatric Obesity: Pediatric Hyperglycemic Hyperosmolar Syndrome," *Pediatric Critical Care Medicine* 6 (2005), 20–24.

xxi   *cancer death rates in the United States fell...* Amanda Gardner, "Cancer Death Rates Still Declining," *Washington Post,* February 20, 2008, *www .washingtonpost.com/wp-dyn/content/article/2008/02/20/AR2008022000995. html.* (Accessed on July 19, 2009.)

xxi   *Heart disease death rates fell...* Steve Sternberg, "Heart Disease Deaths Plummet Ahead of 2010 Goal," *USA Today,* January 22, 2008, *www*

.usatoday.com/news/health/2008-01-22-heart-disease_N.htm. (Accessed on July 19, 2009.)

xxi *Americans aged 70 and over with dementia...* Charles Bankhead, "Decline in Prevalence of Cognitive Impairment Documented," February 20, 2008, *MedPage Today, www.medpagetoday.com/Neurology/Dementia/8427*. (Accessed on July 19, 2009.)

xxi *diabetes was called a pandemic...* K. M. Venkat Narayan, Ping Zhang, Alka M. Kanaya, et al., "Diabetes: The Pandemic and Potential Solutions," in *Disease Control Priorities in Developing Countries*, 2nd edition (New York: Oxford University Press, 2006), 591–604.

xxi *According to Takashi Kadowaki...* He and other international authorities quoted here presented these statistics at the 1st World Congress on Interventional Therapies for Type 2 Diabetes, New York, September 15–16, 2008.

xxii *Even in rural Africa...* Ayesha A. Motala, Tonya Esterhuizen, Eleanor Gouws, et al., "Diabetes Mellitus and Other Disorders of Glycaemia in a Rural South African Community: Prevalence and Associated Risk Factors," *Diabetes Care* 31, no. 9 (September 2008), 1783–88.

CHAPTER 1: PISSING EVIL

Page

3 *Hippocrates... made no mention...* See N. S. Papspyros, *The History of Diabetes Mellitus* (Stuttgart: Georg Thieme Verlag, 1964).

3 *Galen...* Rudolph E. Siegel, *Galen: On the Affected Parts, Translation from the Greek Text with Explanatory Notes* (Basel: S. Karger, 1976), 175.

3 *an Egyptian medical text...* Stephen Carpenter, Michel Rigaud, Mary Barile, et al., *An Interlinear Transliteration and English Translation of Portions of The Ebers Papyrus, Possibly Having to Do with Diabetes Mellitus* (Annandale-on-Hudson, NY: Bard College, 1998).

4 *Aretaeus of Cappadocia...* Aretaeus of Cappadocia, *Of the Causes and Signs of Acute and Chronic Disease*, translated by T. F. Reynolds (London: William Pickering, 1837). Reprinted in *Diabetes: A Medical Odyssey* (Tuckahoe, NY: USV Pharmaceutical Corp., 1971), 1–6.

5 *a Sanskrit medical text...* Kaviraj Kunjalal Bhishagratna, *An English Translation of the Sushruta Samhita*, Based on Original Sanskrit Text (Calcutta, 1907–1916), 27–29; 42–51; 381–91.

5 *Thomas Willis offered treatments...* Thomas Willis, *Pharmaceutice Rationalis* (London: T. Dring, C. Harper and J. Leigh, 1679). Reprinted in *Diabetes: A Medical Odyssey* (Tuckahoe, NY: USV Pharmaceutical Corp., 1971), 7–22.

6 *the physician John Rollo wrote...* John Rollo, *Cases of the Diabetes Mellitus* (London: C. Dilly, 1798). Reprinted in *Diabetes: A Medical Odyssey* (Tuckahoe, NY: USV Pharmaceutical Corp., 1971), 23–44.

7 *New York surgeon Valentine Mott published...* Valentine Mott, "An Account of an Extraordinary Case of Diabetes Mellitus," *American Medical and Philosophical Register*, New York, 1810. Reprinted in *Diabetes: A Medical Odyssey* (Tuckahoe, NY: USV Pharmaceutical Corp., 1971), 45–54.

9 *In 1866... New York City's death rate from diabetes...* This figure is attributed to New York City's Commissioner of Public Health, Haven Emerson. See Mary Ross, "Life Lengthened by Health Work," *New York Times*, August 1, 1926, page X6.

9 *Charles B. Brigham wrote...* Charles B. Brigham, *An Essay Upon Diabetes Mellitus* (Boston: Press of Abner A. Kingman, 1868). Reprinted in *Diabetes: A Medical Odyssey* (Tuckahoe, NY: USV Pharmaceutical Corp., 1971), 71–107.

10 *Oskar Minkowski and Joseph von Mering...* Michael Bliss, *The Discovery of Insulin* (Chicago: University of Chicago Press, 1982), 26. See also Joseph von Mering and Oskar Minkowski, "Diabetes Mellitus After Pancreas Extirpation," *Archiv für Experimentale Pathologie und Pharmacologie* 26 (1889). Translated by Hanna Angel. Reprinted in *Diabetes: A Medical Odyssey* (Tuckahoe, NY: USV Pharmaceutical Corp., 1971), 109–127.

10 *Frederick M. Allen began work...* Michael Bliss, *The Discovery of Insulin* (Chicago: University of Chicago Press, 1982), 33–44.

11 *according to a 1920 report...* Thomas W. Edgar, "The Limitation of Starvation in Diabetes Mellitus," *New York Medical Journal* 61, no. 19 (May 1920), 803–806.

11 *"Individualizing is one of the mainstays"...* Henry S. Stark, "The Drugless Therapy of Diabetes," *New York Medical Journal* 61, no. 19 (May 1920), 800–803.

11 *Betty Crocker invented...* *www.generalmills.com/corporate/company/hist_ betty.pdf.* (Accessed on August 3, 2009.)

12 *by 1900 the toll had reached 10 of every 100,000...* "City Death Rate Up 5 Per Cent in 1926," *New York Times*, March 2, 1927, page 16.

12 *A decade later...* Ibid.

12 *By 1923, it stood at 22.9 per 100,000...* "Mary Ross: Life Lengthened by Health Work," *New York Times*, August 1, 1926, page X6.

12 *According to Dr. Haven Emerson...* Ibid.

12 *Japanese emperor Yoshihito...* Associated Press, "Mikado Forced to Rest," *New York Times*, May 23, 1920, page E1.

13 *"Big Bill" Haywood...* "Says Haywood Is on Joy Ride Before Death," *New York Times*, May 4, 1921, page 23.

13   *Charles M. Schwab's 57-year-old brother...* "Joseph E. Schwab Dies After Long Illness," *New York Times*, February 18, 1922, page 11.

13   *an Italian doctor's claim...* "Consumption Cure Found by Italian?" *New York Times*, June 30, 1918, page 32.

13   *"Insanity Due to Infected Teeth"...* "Finds Insanity Due to Infected Teeth," *New York Times,* October 23, 1918, page 10.

13   *curing diabetes with a kind of bacterium found in yogurt...* "Metchnitkoff Cure for Dread Diabetes Announced," *New York Times*, July 14, 1912, page SM3. "New Diabetes Cure Perfected Here," *New York Times*, July 15, 1912, page 6. "Diabetes Treatment Confirmed by Treatment of 176 Cases," *New York Times*, July 20, 1913, page SM5.

13   *curing it with baking soda...* "Diabetes Cure Announced," *New York Times*, October 10, 1915, page 21.

13   *in despair, drinking himself to bed every night...* As mentioned in the text, much of my account of the discovery of insulin is based on Michael Bliss's book *The Discovery of Insulin*, published in 1982 by the University of Chicago Press. Additional information was obtained from an article by J. J. R. Macleod, "History of the Researches Leading to the Discovery of Insulin," *Bulletin of the History of Medicine* 52, no. 3 (1978): 295–312.

18   *By late November, they submitted a paper...* Frederick G. Banting and Charles H. Best, "The Internal Secretion of the Pancreas," *Journal of Laboratory and Clinical Medicine* 7, no. 5 (February 1922).

20   *Banting appeared on the cover...* *Time: The Weekly News-Magazine* 1, no. 26 (August 27, 1923).

20   *Dr. Joseph Collins published an article...* "Joseph Collins: Diabetes, Dreaded Disease, Yields to New Gland Cure," *New York Times*, May 6, 1923, page XX12.

CHAPTER 2: TWO STEPS BACK

Page

23   *In his speech on "The Story of Insulin"...* "Warns Idle Fail Rapidly in Health," *New York Times*, April 6, 1933, page 20.

23   *By 1926, it reached 25 per 100,000...* "City Death Rate Up 5 Per Cent. in 1926," *New York Times*, March 2, 1927, page 16.

23   *reaching 29 deaths due to diabetes per 100,000 New Yorkers in 1932...* "Diabetes Mortality Up 58% in 30 Years," *New York Times*, April 30, 1933, page 24. "Toll of Diabetes Is Rising Rapidly," *New York Times*, June 22, 1929, page 9.

24 *average life expectancy of New York City residents had in fact jumped...* Mary Ross, "Life Lengthened by Health Work," *New York Times*, August 1, 1926, page X6.

24 *According to the Statistical Bulletin of the Metropolitan Life Insurance Company...* "Toll of Diabetes Is Rising Rapidly," *New York Times*, June 22, 1929, page 9.

24 *Four years later, a study conducted by Godias J. Drolet...* "Diabetes Mortality Up 58% in 30 Years," *New York Times*, April 30, 1933, page 24.

25 *56-year-old Russell Foote...* "Invalid Attempts Suicide; Diabetes Sufferer's Wounds Heal, But He Dies of His Malady," *New York Times*, November 6, 1924, page 20.

26 *others required 200 units or more...* W. S. Lane, E. K. Cochran, and J. A. Jackson, "High-Dose Insulin Therapy: Is It Time for U-500 Insulin?" *Endocrine Practice* 15, no. 1 (January–February 2009): 71–79.

26 *even 1,700 units of insulin were necessary...* B. J. Yauger, P. Gorden, and J. Park, "Effect of Depot Medroxyprogesterone Acetate on Glucose Tolerance in Generalized Lipodystrophy," *Obstetrics and Gynecology* 112, Part 2 (August 2008): 445–47.

26 *Wilhelm Falta, published a paper...* W. Falta and R. Boller, "Insularer und Insulinresistenter Diabetes," *Klin. Wochenschr.* 10 (1931): 438–43.

26 *Falta's observations were confirmed and extended...* Richard Himsworth, "Sir Harold Himsworth MD FRS (1905–1993)," *Diabetologia*, March 2005, *www .diabetologia-journal.org/webpages/covers/2005/march.html*. (Accessed on July 22, 2009.)

27 *the January 18, 1936 edition, of* The Lancet... H. P. Himsworth, "Diabetes Mellitus: Its Differentiation into Insulin-Sensitive and Insulin-Insensitive Types, *Lancet* 1 (January 18, 1936): 127–30.

29 *from 29 per 100,000...* "Diabetes Mortality Up 58% in 30 Years," *New York Times*, April 30, 1933, page 24.

29 *36.2 in January of 1936...* "Deaths in State Near Low Record," *New York Times*, March 23, 1936, page 15.

29 *38.8 for the full year of 1939...* "Good Health Year Enjoyed by City," *New York Times*, January 1, 1940, page 25.

29 *just gluttons...* "Hits Diabetes Statistics; Michigan Professor Says Half the Cases Are 'Just Fatties,'" *New York Times*, September 23, 1938, page 29.

29 *microscopic damage to the kidneys had been observed...* Paul Kimmelstiel and Clifford Wilson, "Intercapillary Lesions in the Glomeruli of the Kidney," *American Journal of Pathology* 12 (January 1936): 83–98.

30 *it took until 1951 for two doctors at Elliott Joslin's clinic...* James Lee Wilson, Howard F. Root, and Alexander Marble, "Diabetic Nephropathy, a Clinical Syndrome," *New England Journal of Medicine* 245, no. 14 (October 4, 1951): 513–17.

32 *Herman O. Mosenthal, took the stage...* American Diabetes Association, *The Journey and the Dream: A History of the American Diabetes Association.* (Alexandria, VA: American Diabetes Association, 1990), 15–16.

32 *Tolstoi wrote in 1948...* Edward Tolstoi, "The Objectives of Modern Diabetic Care," *Psychosomatic Medicine* 10, no. 5 (September–October 1948): 291–94.

33 *170,469 tiny new residents...* "Births Set Record in the City for '47," *New York Times,* January 1, 1948, page 25.

33 *death rate due to diabetes hit a new high, 44.4 per 100,000...* Ibid.

33 *Hans Hagedorn, had an idea...* Walter Sneader, *Drug Discovery: A History* (Chichester, England: John Wiley and Sons, 2005), 167.

34 *September of 1936, when Elliott Joslin was invited to speak...* William L. Laurence, "Improved Insulin Aids in Diabetes," *New York Times,* September 15, 1936, page 16.

34 *study presented in Denver at the June 1937 meeting...* Associated Press, "Obesity Is Linked to Blood Control; Two California Scientists Experiment with Protamine Zinc Insulin on Rats," *New York Times,* June 22, 1937, page 25.

34 *As early as 1926, researchers in Minkowski's laboratory...* See Herbert Hirsch-Kauffman, "Synthalin B," *American Journal of Diseases of Children* 41, no. 4 (1931): 1004. See also Walter Sneader, *Drug Prototypes and Their Exploitation* (New York: John Wiley, 1996), 736.

35 *synthalin's brief flirtation with the European market ended...* Jeremy A. Greene, *Prescribing by Numbers: Drugs and the Definition of Disease* (Baltimore: Johns Hopkins University Press, 2007), 88.

35 *The first true breakthrough in the search for a pill...* For my account of how Orinase and other sulfonylureas were developed and marketed, and how the medical community reacted in the 1970s to the UGDP study, I have drawn generously upon Jeremy A. Greene's extraordinary book, cited in full above, *Prescribing by Numbers.* Dr. Greene, an assistant professor in the department of the History of Science at Harvard University, also spoke with me about this subject. I recommend his book to anyone interested in the fascinating history of how minimally useful drugs become blockbusters.

37 *Seymour L. Shapiro, a chemist at the company...* I stumbled upon the forgotten role of Dr. Shapiro in the dedication to *Diabetes: A Medical Odyssey* (Tuckahoe, NY: USV Pharmaceutical Corp., 1971). With virtually no other published accounts of Dr. Shapiro's work to go on, I was lucky enough to track down and interview Harvey S. Sadow, PhD, the clinical pharmacologist at USV who worked with Shapiro and led the effort to establish the clinical usefulness of phenformin. "The sad thing," Dr. Sadow told me, "was that Seymour Shapiro died before he could take a bow for his work." Even though phenformin is no longer sold in the United States, its development by Dr. Shapiro and others at USV can be fairly said to have paved the way for metformin, a chemical cousin that is now among the mostly widely used, and most useful, drugs for type 2.

38 *2 million people with diabetes in 1960...* American Diabetes Association, *The Journey and the Dream: A History of the American Diabetes Association* (Alexandria, VA: American Diabetes Association, 1990), 102.

38 *2.3 million in 1965, or 12.2 per thousand...* Ibid., page 123.

38 *a longer article about the study appeared in the* Washington Post... Morton Mintz, "Antidiabetes Pill Held Causing Early Death," *Washington Post*, May 21, 1970.

41 *A new, more liberal diet was approved by the ADA...* American Diabetes Association, *The Journey and the Dream: A History of the American Diabetes Association* (Alexandria, VA: American Diabetes Association, 1990), 197–200.

41 *The chemical structure of insulin was fully synthesized...* Reuters, "Swiss Drug Concern Reports a Synthesis of Human Insulin," *New York Times*, December 21, 1974, page 7.

41 *Lasers were studied...* Harold M. Schmeck Jr., "Light Beam Treatments Reduce Diabetic Blindness," *New York Times*, April 2, 1976, page 24.

41 *first transplants of insulin-producing islet cells...* J. S. Najarian, D. E. R. Sutherland, A. T. Matas, et al., "Human Islet Transplantation: A Preliminary Report," *Transplantation Proceedings* 9: 233–36.

41 *National Commission on Diabetes...* Harold M. Schmeck Jr., "Diabetes Rated 3d Killer; U.S. Panel Calls for Help," *New York Times*, December 11, 1975, page 93.

42 *Jackie Robinson had died of complications of the disease...* Lawrence K. Altman, "Diabetes Called Basic Cause of Robinson's Death," *New York Times*, October 29, 1972, page 61.

42 *Walt Kelly...died of it in 1973...* "Walt Kelly, Pogo Creator, Dies," *New York Times*, October 19, 1973, page 46.

CHAPTER 3: TRY HARDER

Page

46 *Back in 1976, researchers had reported on a blood test...* Bayer Webster, "New Tests Found to Fight Diabetes," *New York Times*, August 19, 1976, page 16.

48 *Diabetes Control and Complications Trial...* Dan Hurley, "Tight Glycemic Control Urged for All Diabetics," *Medical Tribune* 34, no. 13 (July 8, 1993): 1.

51 *fewer than 6,000 board-certified endocrinologists...* Endocrine Society, "U.S. Endocrinology Workforce Shortage Represents Significant Threat to Public Health," January 30, 2008, *www.endo-society.org/media/press/2008/Endocrinology-Workforce-Shortage-Represents.cfm.* (Accessed on July 26, 2009.)

52 *primitive insulin pumps had been around since the late 1970s...* W. M. Tamborlane, R. S. Sherwin, and M. Genel, et al., "Reduction to Normal of Plasma Glucose in Juvenile Diabetes by Subcutaneous Administration of Insulin with a Portable Infusion Pump," *New England Journal of Medicine* 300, no. 11 (March 15, 1979): 573–78.

53 *on August 10, 2005, the FDA finally approved...* "Medtronic Announces FDA Approval of Real-Time Continuous Glucose Monitoring System," *www.oes.org/page2/4456~Approval_Of_Medtronics_Real-Time_Continuous_Glucose_Monitor.html.* (Accessed on July 26, 2009.)

53 *I managed to convince my editor...* The resulting article appeared in the *New York Times* on August 29, 2006, under the headline "The Beep of the Sensor, the Thrill of Control."

56 *depression is twice as common...* Jill Stein, "Adult Type 1 Diabetics Have Higher Depression Rates," Reuters Health, June 8, 2009, *www.nlm.nih.gov/medlineplus/news/fullstory_85378.html.* (Accessed on July 26, 2009.)

57 *30 percent of young women engage in such behaviors...* Ann E. Goebel-Fabbri, Janna Fikkan, Debra L. Franko, et al., "Insulin Restriction and Associated Morbidity and Mortality in Women with Type 1 Diabetes," *Diabetes Care* 31 (March 2008): 415–19.

58 *in June of 2000, a major breakthrough was reported...* A. M. James Shapiro, Jonathan R. T. Lakey, Edmond A. Ryan, et al., "Islet Transplantation in Seven Patients with Type 1 Diabetes Mellitus Using a Glucocorticoid-Free Immunosuppressive Regimen," *New England Journal of Medicine* 343, no. 4 (July 27, 2000): 230–38.

59 *Even* The New Yorker *published an article...* Jerome Groopman, "The Edmonton Protocol," *The New Yorker*, February 10, 2003, page 48.

59 *"Diabetes Treatment Fails to Live Up to Promise"...* Denise Grady, "Diabetes Treatment Fails to Live Up to Promise," *New York Times*, September 28,

2006, *www.nytimes.com/2006/09/28/health/28diabetes.html*. (Accessed on July 26, 2009.)

60   *variations in certain genes that code for the immune system...* D. P. Singal and M. A. Blajchman, "Histocompatibility (HL-A) Antigens, Lymphocytotoxic Antibodies and Tissue Antibodies in Patients with Diabetes Mellitus," *Diabetes* 22 (1973): 429–32. See also J. Nerup, P. Platz, O. O. Anderssen, et al., "HL-A Antigens and Diabetes Mellitus," *Lancet* 12, no. 2 (1974): 864–66.

60   *if white blood cells from people with type 1 diabetes were placed in a test tube with islet cells...* G. F. Bottazzo, A. Florin-Christensen, and D. Doniach, "Islet Cell Antibodies in Diabetes Mellitus with Autoimmune Polyendocrine Deficiencies," *Lancet* 2, no. 7892 (November 1974): 1279–83. See also A. C. MacCuish, E. W. Barnes, W. J. Irvine, et al., "Antibodies to Pancreatic Islet-Cells in Insulin-Dependent Diabetics with Coexistent Autoimmune Disease," *Lancet* 2, no. 7896 (December 28, 1974): 1529–31.

60   *predict with 50 percent to 90 percent accuracy their likelihood of developing type 1...* Abner Louis Notkins and Åke Lernmark, "Autoimmune Type 1 Diabetes: Resolved and Unresolved Issues," *Journal of Clinical Investigation* 108, no. 9 (November 2001): 1247–52.

61   *"The Rise of Childhood Type 1"...* Edwin A. M. Gale, "The Rise of Childhood Type 1 Diabetes in the 20th Century," *Diabetes* 51, no. 12 (December 2002): 3353–61.

61   *the yearly incidence of new cases of type 1 had jumped to 14.8 per 100,000 children in Colorado...* Kendra Vehik, Richard F. Hamman, Dennis Lezotte, et al., "Increasing Incidence of Type 1 Diabetes in 0- to 17-Year-Old Colorado Youth," *Diabetes Care* 30, no. 3 (March 2007): 503–509.

61   *By the opening years of the 21st century...* Ronny A. Bell, Elizabeth J. Mayer-Davis, Jennifer W. Beyer, et al., "Diabetes in Non-Hispanic White Youth: Prevalence, Incidence, and Clinical Characteristics: The SEARCH for Diabetes in Youth Study," *Diabetes Care* 32 (2009): S102–S111.

62   *a 2007 editorial in the* Journal of the American Medical Association... Rebecca B. Lipton, "Incidence of Diabetes in Children and Youth—Tracking a Moving Target," *Journal of the American Medical Association* 298, no. 24 (June 2007): 2760–62.

CHAPTER 4: THE SWEETEST PLACE ON EARTH

Page

65   *Buffalo Creek had been the site of a notorious disaster...* West Virginia Division of Culture and History, Buffalo Creek, *www.wvculture.org/hiStory/buffcreek/bctitle.html*. (Accessed on July 27, 2009.) Also see George Vecsey,

"Miners Cling to Homes That Are Left After Flood," *New York Times*, March 1, 1972, page 23.

69   *Orinase and other sulfonylureas were required by the FDA...* See Jeremy A. Greene, *Prescribing by Numbers: Drugs and the Definition of Disease* (Baltimore: Johns Hopkins University Press, 2007): 144.

70   *The next big drug to hit the market, Rezulin...* The story of how the FDA rushed through the approval of Rezulin, and then delayed withdrawing it from the market after its risks had been established, was highlighted in a Pulitzer prize–winning series (for investigative reporting, 2001) in the *Los Angeles Times* by reporter David Willman, beginning on February 19, 2000, with "Key Physician Urges Rezulin Be Withdrawn." The articles include March 10, 2000, "Fears Grow Over Delay in Removing Rezulin"; March 17, 2000, "Physician Who Opposes Rezulin Is Threatened by FDA With Dismissal"; March 22, 2000, "Diabetes Drug Rezulin Pulled Off the Market"; August 16, 2000, "FDA's Approval and Delay in Withdrawing Rezulin Probed"; and December 20, 2000, "New FDA: How a New Policy Led to 7 Deadly Drugs." These and other pieces in the series are gathered at *www .pulitzer.org/works/2001-Investigative-Reporting.* (Accessed on July 28, 2009.)

71   *Steven Nissen...published an analysis...* Steven E. Nissen and Kathy Wolski, "Effect of Rosiglitazone on the Risk of Myocardial Infarction and Death from Cardiovascular Causes," *New England Journal of Medicine* 356, no. 24 (May 14, 2007): 2457–71.

72   *Action to Control Cardiovascular Risk in Diabetes (ACCORD) study...* "The Action to Control Cardiovascular Risk in Diabetes Study Group: Effects of Intensive Glucose Lowering in Type 2 Diabetes," *New England Journal of Medicine* 358, no. 24 (June 12, 2008): 2545–59.

72   *"confusing and disturbing"...* Gina Kolata, "Diabetes Study Partially Halted After Deaths," *New York Times*, February 7, 2008.

72   *another large study, known as ADVANCE...* The ADVANCE Collaborative Group, "Intensive Blood Glucose Control and Vascular Outcomes in Patients with Type 2 Diabetes," *New England Journal of Medicine* 358, no. 24 (June 12, 2008): 2560–72.

73   *Veterans Affairs Diabetes Trial...* William Duckworth, Carlos Abraira, Thomas Moritz, et al., "Glucose Control and Vascular Complications in Veterans with Type 2 Diabetes," *New England Journal of Medicine* 360, no. 2 (January 8, 2009): 129–39.

73   *United Kingdom Prospective Diabetes Study...* Rury R. Holman, Sanjoy K. Paul, M. Angelyn Bethel, et al., "10-Year Follow-up of Intensive Glucose Control in Type 2 Diabetes," *New England Journal of Medicine* 359, no. 15 (October 9, 2008): 1577–89.

73 *the FDA scheduled a meeting of its diabetes drug advisory committee...* Complete transcripts of the meeting on July 1 and 2, 2008, can be found on the FDA website at *www.fda.gov/ohrms/dockets/AC/cder08.html#Endocrinologic Metabolic.* (Accessed on July 28, 2009.)

75 *In 2001, the largest study ever conducted to test the ability of diet and exercise to* prevent *diabetes...* W. C. Knowler, E. Barrett-Connor, S. E. Fowler, et al., "Reduction in the Incidence of Type 2 Diabetes with Lifestyle Intervention or Metformin," *New England Journal of Medicine* 346, no. 6 (February 7, 2002): 393–403.

75 *As Nathan told the* New York Times... Kenneth Chang, "Diet and Exercise Are Found to Cut Diabetes by Over Half," *New York Times*, August 9, 2001.

75 *By 2001, the year Dr. Nathan's lifestyle study was released, the figure had reached 16 million...* Ibid.

75 *23.6 million in 2009...* Centers for Disease Control and Prevention, 2007 National Diabetes Fact Sheet, *www.cdc.gov/diabetes/pubs/estimates07.htm.* (Accessed on July 28, 2009.)

76 *according to the CDC, diabetes remains the leading cause...* Ibid.

77 *CDC released county-by-county breakdowns...* Centers for Disease Control and Prevention, County Level Estimates of Diagnosed Diabetes—U.S. Maps, *http://apps.nccd.cdc.gov/DDT_STRS2/NationalDiabetesPrevalenceEstimates. aspx.* (Accessed on July 28, 2009.)

77 *average lifespan of women in Logan County actually* dropped... Eric Eyre, "Life Short for W.Va. Women," *Charleston Gazette*, September 5, 2008, *http://wvcc.org/docs/InTheNews/EarlyDeathsWVGazette.html.* (Accessed on July 28, 2009.)

78 *website of the one hospital in the county...* www.loganregionalmedicalcenter. net/. (Accessed on July 28, 2009.)

CHAPTER 5: THE ACCELERATOR HYPOTHESIS

Page

93 *Wilkin's first paper on the subject...* Terry Wilkin, "The Primary Lesion Theory of Autoimmunity: A Speculative Hypothesis," *Autoimmunity* 7, no. 4 (1990): 225–35.

93 *a pro-and-con pair of articles...* Terry Wilkin, "Pro: Evidence for a Primary Lesion in the Target Organ in Autoimmune Disease," *International Archives of Allergy and Immunology* 103, no. 4 (1994): 323–27. H. Wekerle, H. Lassmann, "Contra: Evidence Against a Primary Lesion in the Target Organ in Autoimmune Disease," *International Archives of Allergy and Immunology* 103, no. 4 (1994): 328–31.

94 *First set in print in July of 2001...* T. J. Wilkin, "The Accelerator Hypothesis: Weight Gain as the Missing Link Between Type I and Type II Diabetes," *Diabetologia* 44, no. 7 (2001): 914–22.

96 *In Britain, a 2003 study led by Wilkin...* M. Kibirige, B. Metcalf, R. Renuka, et al., "Testing the Accelerator Hypothesis: The Relationship Between Body Mass and Age at Diagnosis of Type 1 Diabetes," *Diabetes Care* 26 (2003): 2865–70.

96 *In Germany and Austria, a 2005 study...* I. Knerr, J. Wolf, R. Reinehr, et al., "The 'Accelerator Hypothesis': Relationship Between Weight, Height, Body Mass Index and Age at Diagnosis in a Large Cohort of 9,248 German and Austrian Children with Type 1 Diabetes Mellitus," *Diabetologia* 48 (2005): 2501–2504.

96 *In Sweden, a 2008 study...* M. Ljungkrantz, J. Ludvigsson, and U. Samuelsson, "Type 1 Diabetes: Increased Height and Weight Gains in Early Childhood," *Pediatric Diabetes* 9, no. 3, part 2 (June 2008): 50–56.

96 *In Australia, a study published in January of 2009...* Jennifer J. Couper and Sarah Beresford, "Weight Gain in Early Life Predicts Risk of Islet Auto-immunity in Children with a First-Degree Relative with Type 1 Diabetes," *Diabetes Care* 32, no. 1 (January 2009): 94–99.

97 *Swedish researchers reported in 2002...* G. Kaati, L. O. Bygren, and S. Edvinsson, "Cardiovascular and Diabetes Mortality Determined by Nutrition During Parents' and Grandparents' Slow Growth Period," *European Journal of Human Genetics* 10 (2002): 682–88.

97 *published in* Diabetologia *in 2004...* S. Fourlanos, P. Narendran, and G. B. Byrnes, "Insulin Resistance Is a Risk Factor for Progression to Type 1 Diabetes," *Diabetologia* 47, no. 10 (2004): 1661–67.

98 *Two other studies have reached the same conclusion...* P. Xu, D. Cuthbertson, and C. Greenbaum, "Role of Insulin Resistance in Predicting Progression to Type 1 Diabetes," *Diabetes Care* 30, no. 9 (September 2007), 2314–20. P. J. Bingley, J. L. Mahon, and E. A. M. Gale, "Insulin Resistance and Progression to Type 1 Diabetes in the European Nicotinamide Diabetes Intervention Trial (ENDIT)," *Diabetes Care* 31, no. 1 (January 2008): 146–50.

98 *a 2001 study from the Cleveland Clinic Foundation...* Y. Z. Grasso, S. K. Reddy, C. R. Rosenfeld, et al., "Autoantibodies to IA-2 and GAD65 in Patients with Type 2 Diabetes Mellitus of Varied Duration: Prevalence and Correlation with Clinical Features," *Endocrine Practice* 7, no. 5 (September–October 2001): 339–45.

102 *One of the papers even found...* Jian Liu, Adeline Divoux, Jiusong Sun, et al., "Genetic Deficiency and Pharmacological Stabilization of Mast Cells Reduce Diet-Induced Obesity and Diabetes in Mice," *Nature Medicine.* Published online July 26, 2009, prior to print, *www.nature.com/nm/journal/vaop/ncurrent/full/nm.1994.html.* (Accessed August 4, 2009.)

103 *Back in 1989, she told the British newspaper...* Bonnie Siegler, "Halle Berry: My Battle with Diabetes," *Daily Mail*, December 14, 2005, *www.dailymail.co.uk/ health/article-371528/Halle-Berry-My-battle-diabetes.html*. (Accessed on July 28, 2009.)

104 *in an interview with the website contactmusic.com in October of 2007...* www .contactmusic.com/news.nsf/article/berry%20beating%20diabetes_1048407. (Accessed on July 28, 2009.)

104 *ABC NEWS.com opened its article...* Russell Goldman, "Berry's Miracle Cure Probably Misdiagnosis, Say Docs," November 6, 2007, *www.abcnews.go.com/ Health/story?id=3822870&page=1*. (Accessed on July 28, 2009.)

104 *"insane" and "moronic"...* Kelly Kunik, "So, Back to the Madness that Is and Was Caused by Halle Berry," *Diabetesaliciousness*, November 14, 2007, *http://diabetesaliciousness.blogspot.com/2007/11/so-back-to-madness-that-is-and-was.html*. (Accessed on July 28, 2009.)

105 *One of the most balanced views on Wilkin's hypothesis...* Edwin A. M. Gale, "To Boldly Go—or to Go Too Boldly? The Accelerator Hypothesis Revisited," *Diabetologia* 50, no. 8 (August 2007): 1571–75.

105 *ethnic Finns who live in the western portion of Russia...* A. Kondrashova, A. Reunanen, and A. Romanov, "A Six-fold Gradient in the Incidence of Type 1 Diabetes at the Eastern Border of Finland," *Annals of Medicine* 37, no. 1 (2005): 67–72.

106 *As Poland's economy took off...* P. Jarosz-Chobot, J. Polanska, and A. Polanski, "Does Social-Economical Transformation Influence the Incidence of Type 1 Diabetes Mellitus? A Polish Example," *Pediatric Diabetes* 9, no. 3, part 1 (June 2008): 202–207.

106 *A 2001 paper in* Diabetologia *even went so far...* C. C. Patterson, G. Dahlquist, and G. Soltész, "Is Childhood-Onset Type I Diabetes a Wealth-Related Disease? An Ecological Analysis of European Incidence Rates," *Diabetologia* 44, Suppl. 3 (October 2001): B9–B16.

CHAPTER 6. THE COW'S MILK HYPOTHESIS

Page

110 *Martin had published a trail-blazing study...* R. B. Elliott and J. M. Martin, "Dietary Protein: A Trigger of Insulin-Dependent Diabetes in the BB Rat?" *Diabetologia* 26 (1984): 297–99.

111 *The work had led to important papers on the functioning of T cells...* A. Shore, S. Limatibul, H. M. Dosch, et al., "Identification of Two Serum Components Regulating the Expression of T-Lymphocyte Function in Childhood Myasthenia Gravis," *New England Journal of Medicine* 301, no. 12 (September 20,

1979): 625–29. H. M. Dosch, A. Mansour, A. Cohen, et al., "Inhibition of Suppressor T-Cell Development Following Deoxyguanosine Administration," *Nature* 285, no. 5765 (June 12, 1980): 494–96.

113 *a study published that very month...* L. Blom, G. Dahlquist, and L. Nyström, "The Swedish Childhood Diabetes Study—Social and Perinatal Determinants for Diabetes in Childhood," *Diabetologia* 32, no. 1 (January 1989): 7–13.

113 *Åkerblom and his colleagues had recently discovered...* E. Savilahti, H. K. Åkerblom, and V. M. Tainio, "Children with Newly Diagnosed Insulin Dependent Diabetes Mellitus Have Increased Levels of Cow's Milk Antibodies," *Diabetes Research* 7, no. 3 (March 1988): 137–40.

113 *international variations in per-capita consumption of milk correlated well...* K. Dahl-Jørgensen, G. Joner, and K. F. Hanssen, "Relationship between Cows' Milk Consumption and Incidence of IDDM in Childhood," *Diabetes Care* 14, no. 11 (November 1991): 1081–83.

116 *In the July 30, 1992, edition...* J. Karjalainen, J. M. Martin, and M. Knip, "A Bovine Albumin Peptide as a Possible Trigger of Insulin-Dependent Diabetes Mellitus," *New England Journal of Medicine* 327, no. 5: 302–307.

116 *one in the* New York Times, *quoting him as saying...* Warren E. Leary, "Protein in Cow Milk May Set Off Juvenile Diabetes," *New York Times,* July 30, 1992.

117 *A more serious attack came in December of 1993...* M. A. Atkinson, M. A. Bowman, K. J. Kao, et al., "Lack of Immune Responsiveness to Bovine Serum Albumin in Insulin-Dependent Diabetes," *New England Journal of Medicine* 329 (1993): 1853–58.

117 *Dosch and colleagues fired back...* H. M. Dosch, J. Karjalainen, J. Vander-Meulen, et al., "Lack of Immunity to Bovine Serum Albumin in Insulin-Dependent Diabetes Mellitus," *New England Journal of Medicine* 330 (1994): 1616–17.

121 *Soluble Food for Babies...* Harvey Levenstein, *Revolution at the Table: The Transformation of the American Diet* (New York: Oxford University Press, 1988): 122–23. See also Lynne Olver, Food Timeline FAQs: Baby Food, *www .foodtimeline.org/foodbaby.html.*

121 *by the early 1960s fully 90 percent were on the bottle...* Joan Beck, "Feeding a Baby Is Easier, but There Are Still Problems," *Chicago Tribune,* March 24, 1964, page A2.

122 *"breastfeeding rates among young infants are discouragingly low"...* Anne Merewood, Reginald Fonrose, Marcella Singleton, et al., "From Maine to Mississippi: Hospital Distribution of Formula Sample Packs Along the Eastern Seaboard," *Archives of Pediatric Adolescence Medicine* 162, no. 9 (2008): 823–27.

123 *In 2008, Knip reported...* Mikael Knip, *TRIGR—The Second Pilot Study*, European Association for the Study of Diabetes, 2008.

123 *Trial to Reduce IDDM (Insulin Dependent Diabetes Mellitus) in the Genetically at Risk, or TRIGR...* For more information on TRIGR, see *http://trigr. epi.usf.edu/*.

CHAPTER 7. THE POP HYPOTHESIS

Page

127 *Woburn became nationally known...* Jonathan Harr, *A Civil Action* (New York: Random House, 1995).

127 *Leukemia diagnosed in over two dozen kids there...* See also "Science in the Courtroom: The Woburn Toxic Trial," at *http://serc.carleton.edu/woburn/ index.html*. (Accessed on July 29, 2009.)

130 *Mayor John C. Curran requested...* Maureen Costello, "Some Suspect School Building in Student Diabetes Cases; Mayor Asks State to Probe Possible Link," *Boston Globe*, September 26, 2004. A copy of the report by the state department of public health can be found online at *www.mass.gov/Eeohhs2/ docs/dph/.../iaq/.../woburn_ges05a.doc*. (Accessed on July 29, 2009.)

132 *Back in 1973, Arizona physicians observed...* S. J. Goldberg, M. D. Lebowitz, E. J. Graver, et al., "An Association of Human Congenital Cardiac Malformations and Drinking Water Contaminants," *Journal of the American College of Cardiology* 16, no. 1 (July 1990): 155–64.

133 *a 2004 study in the journal* Birth Defects Research... J. S. Yauck, M. E. Malloy, and K. Blair, "Proximity of Residence to Trichloroethylene-Emitting Sites and Increased Risk of Offspring Congenital Heart Defects Among Older Women," *Birth Defects Research* 70, no. 10 (October 2004): 808–814.

133 *a review of the published literature on TCE by the Agency for Toxic Substances and Disease Registry...* Ginger L. Gist and JeAnne R. Burg, "Trichloroethylene—A Review of the Literature in View of the Results of the Trichloroethylene Subregistry Results," *www.atsdr.cdc.gov/NER/TCE/a6rev.html*. (Accessed on July 29, 2009.)

133 *Air Force investigators reported in 1997...* G. L. Henriksen, N. S. Ketchum, and J. E. Michalek, "Serum Dioxin and Diabetes Mellitus in Veterans of Operation Ranch Hand," *Epidemiology* 8, no. 3 (May 1997): 252–58.

134 *A follow-up study, published in 2008...* J. E. Michalek and M. Pavuk, "Diabetes and Cancer in Veterans of Operation Ranch Hand After Adjustment for Calendar Period, Days of Spraying, and Time Spent in Southeast Asia," *Journal of Occupational and Environmental Medicine* 50, no. 3 (March 2008): 330–40.

134 *In 2008, researchers at Taiwan's National Health Research Institutes reported...* S. L. Wang, P. C. Tsai, and C. Y. Yang, "Increased Risk of Diabetes and Polychlorinated Biphenyls and Dioxins: A 24-Year Follow-Up Study of the Yucheng Cohort," *Diabetes Care* 31, no. 8 (August 2008): 1574–79.

134 *In Seveso, Italy...* Dario Consonni, Angela C. Pesatori, Carlo Zocchetti, et al., "Mortality in a Population Exposed to Dioxin after the Seveso, Italy, Accident in 1976: 25 Years of Follow-Up," *American Journal of Epidemiology* 167, no. 7 (2008): 847–58.

134 *On April Fool's Day of 2008...* State University of New York, SUNY Upstate Medical University Collaborates on National Study Linking PCBs and Diabetes, *www.upstate.edu/publicaffairs/update/archive_2008/080514.pdf.* (Accessed on July 29, 2009.)

135 *In 2007, researchers at the University of Albany reported...* N. Codru, M. J. Schymura, S. Negoita, et al., "Diabetes in Relation to Serum Levels of Polychlorinated Biphenyls and Chlorinated Pesticides in Adult Native Americans," *Environmental Health Perspectives* 115, no. 10 (October 2007): 1442–47.

135 *residents living in zip codes containing hazardous waste sites...* M. Kouznetsova, X. Huang, J. Ma, et al., "Increased Rate of Hospitalization for Diabetes and Residential Proximity of Hazardous Waste Sites," *Environmental Health Perspectives* 115, no. 1 (January 2007): 75–79.

136 *Carpenter studied how often a person could safely eat salmon...* X. Huang, R. A. Hites, J. A. Foran, et al., "Consumption Advisories for Salmon Based on Risk of Cancer and Noncancer Health Effects," *Environmental Research* 101, no. 2 (June 2006): 263–74.

137 *In 2003, researchers from Brussels...* S. Fierens, H. Mairesse, J. F. Heilier, et al., "Dioxin/Polychlorinated Biphenyl Body Burden, Diabetes and Endometriosis: Findings in a Population-Based Study in Belgium," *Biomarkers* 8, no. 6 (November–December 2003): 529–34.

137 *a study published in 2006 in the journal* Diabetes Care... Duk-Hee Lee, In-Kyu Lee, Kyungeun Song, et al., "A Strong Dose-Response Relation Between Serum Concentrations of Persistent Organic Pollutants and Diabetes," *Diabetes Care* 29 (2006): 1638–44.

138 *two editorials in the prominent British medical journal...* Miquel Porta, "Persistent Organic Pollutants and the Burden of Diabetes," *Lancet* 368 (August 12, 2006): 558–59. Oliver A. H. Jones, Mahon L. Maguire, and Julian L. Griffin, "Environmental Pollution and Diabetes: A Neglected Association," *Lancet* 371 (January 26, 2008): 287–88.

139 *a study they did involving 4,088 Koreans...* D. H. Lee, J. H. Kim, D. C. Christiani, et al., "Gamma-glutamyltransferase and Diabetes—A 4-Year Follow-up Study," *Diabetologia* 46, no. 3 (March 2003): 359–64.

139 *another study by Lee and Jacobs, involving 8,072 Korean men...* D. H. Lee, M. H. Ha, S. Kam, et al., "A Strong Secular Trend in Serum Gamma-gluta-myltransferase from 1996 to 2003 Among South Korean Men," *American Journal of Epidemiology* 163, no. 1 (January 2006): 57–65.

140 *Longnecker published three papers...* M. P. Longnecker and J. L. Daniels, "Environmental Contaminants as Etiologic Factors for Diabetes," *Environmental Health Perspectives* 109, Supp. 6 (December 2001): 871–76. M. P. Longnecker, M. A. Klebanoff, J. W. Brock, et al., "Polychlorinated Biphenyl Serum Levels in Pregnant Subjects with Diabetes," *Diabetes Care* 24, no. 6 (June 2001): 1099–1101. M. P. Longnecker and J. E. Michalek, "Serum Dioxin Level in Relation to Diabetes Mellitus among Air Force Veterans with Background Levels of Exposure," *Epidemiology* 11, no. 1 (January 2000): 44–48.

142 *in 2008, researchers from Britain and Iowa reported...* I. A. Lang, T. S. Galloway, A. Scarlett, et al., "Association of Urinary Bisphenol A Concentration with Medical Disorders and Laboratory Abnormalities in Adults," *Journal of the American Medical Association* 300, no. 11 (September 2008): 1303–1310.

143 *tests found traces of arsenic in the groundwater there...* Nicholas Scofield, "School Committee Hears Goodyear School Options," February 12, 2009, *www.wickedlocal.com/woburn/homepage/x1450776107/School-Committee-hears-Goodyear-School-options.* (Accessed on July 29, 2009.)

CHAPTER 8: THE SUNSHINE HYPOTHESIS

Page

147 *a study that was published six years later...* C. F. Garland and F. C. Garland, "Do Sunlight and Vitamin D Reduce the Likelihood of Colon Cancer?" *International Journal of Epidemiology* 9, no. 3 (September 1980): 227–31.

147 *In 1985 Cedric co-authored a study...* C. F. Garland, R. B. Shekelle, E. Barrett-Connor, et al., "Dietary Vitamin D and Calcium and Risk of Colorectal Cancer: A 19-Year Prospective Study In Men," *Lancet* 1, no. 8424 (February 9, 1985): 307–309.

148 *The study they published, again in* The Lancet... C. F. Garland, G. W. Comstock, F. C. Garland, et al., "Serum 25-Hydroxyvitamin D and Colon Cancer: Eight-Year Prospective Study," *Lancet* 2, no. 8673 (November 18, 1989): 1176–78.

148 *dramatic reductions in the risk of cardiovascular disease...* See, for instance, Thomas J. Wang, Michael J. Pencina, Sarah L. Booth, et al., "Vitamin D Deficiency and Risk of Cardiovascular Disease," *Circulation* 117 (2008): 453–55.

148 *multiple sclerosis...* See, for instance, Kassandra L. Munger, Lynn I. Levin, Bruce W. Hollis, et al., "Serum 25-Hydroxyvitamin D Levels and Risk of

Multiple Sclerosis," *Journal of the American Medical Association* 296, no. 23 (December 20, 2006): 2832–38.

148 *Alzheimer's disease, Parkinson's disease...* See, for instance, M. L. Evatt, M. R. Delong, N. Khazai, et al., "Prevalence of Vitamin D Insufficiency in Patients with Parkinson Disease and Alzheimer Disease," *Archives of Neurology* 65, no. 10 (October 2008): 1348–52.

148 *schizophrenia...* See, for instance, D. K. Kinney, P. Teixeira, D. Hsu, et al., "Relation of Schizophrenia Prevalence to Latitude, Climate, Fish Consumption, Infant Mortality, and Skin Color: A Role for Prenatal Vitamin D Deficiency and Infections?" *Schizophrenia Bulletin* 35, no. 3 (May 2009): 582–95.

149 *a startling study from Finland...* E. Hyppönen, E. Läärä, A. Reunanen, et al., "Intake of Vitamin D and Risk of Type 1 Diabetes: A Birth-Cohort Study," *Lancet* 358, no. 9292 (November 3, 2001): 1500–1503.

150 *have been linked to decreased insulin* secretion... C. Mathieu, C. Gysemans, and A. Giulietti, "Vitamin D and Diabetes," *Diabetologia* 48, no. 7 (July 2005): 1247–57.

150 *and increased insulin* resistance... N. G. Forouhi, J. Luan, and A. Cooper, "Baseline Serum 25-Hydroxy Vitamin D Is Predictive of Future Glycemic Status and Insulin Resistance," *Diabetes* 57, no. 10 (October 2008): 2619–25.

150 *Perhaps the most powerful study of type 2 and vitamin D...* Anastassios G. Pittas, Bess Dawson-Hughes, and Tricia Li, "Vitamin D and Calcium Intake in Relation to Type 2 Diabetes in Women," *Diabetes Care* 29 (2006): 650–56.

151 *Finland's annual incidence of newly diagnosed cases of type 1 soared...* V. Harjutsalo, L. Sjöberg, and J. Tuomilehto, "Time Trends in the Incidence of Type 1 Diabetes in Finnish Children: A Cohort Study," *Lancet* 371, no. 96260 (May 24, 2008): 1777–82.

151 *In the United States, the minimum recommended daily intake of vitamin D...* Office of Dietary Supplements, National Institutes of Health, Dietary Supplement Fact Sheet: Vitamin D, *http://ods.od.nih.gov/factsheets/vitamind.asp.* (Accessed on July 30, 2009.)

151 *"These findings have important implications"...* Adit A. Ginde, Mark C. Liu, and Carlos A. Camargo Jr., "Demographic Differences and Trends of Vitamin D Insufficiency in the US Population, 1988-2004," *Archives of Internal Medicine* 169, no. 6 (March 2009): 626–32.

151 *seven out of ten children...* Juhi Kumar, Michal L. Melamed, Paul Muntner, et al., "Prevalence and Associations of 25-Hydroxyvitamin D Deficiency in Children and Adolescents in the United States: Results from NHANES 2001–2004," *Pediatrics.* Published online prior to print on August 3, 2009. www.eurekalert.org/pub_releases/2009-08/aeco-mou072909.php

151   videophilia... Oliver Pergams and Patricia Zaradic, "Evidence for a Fundamental and Pervasive Shift Away from Nature-Based Recreation," *Proceedings of the National Academy of Sciences* 105, no. 7 (February 19, 2008): 2295–300.

152   *In sunny spots like Cuba, Peru, and Bermuda...* S. B. Mohr, C. F. Garland, E. D. Gorham, et al., "The Association Between Ultraviolet B Irradiance, Vitamin D Status and Incidence Rates of Type 1 Diabetes in 51 Regions Worldwide," *Diabetologia* 51, no. 8 (August 2008): 1391–98.

152   *"In Boston, you cannot make any vitamin D"...* Natalie Angier, "Sunlight and Breast Cancer: Danger in Darkness?" *New York Times*, December 6, 1990.

154   *The Women's Health Initiative...* A. Z. LaCroix, J. Kotchen, G. Anderson, et al., "Calcium plus Vitamin D Supplementation and Mortality in Postmenopausal Women: The Women's Health Initiative Calcium–Vitamin D Randomized Controlled Trial," *Journals of Gerontology* 64, no. 5 (May 2009): 559–67.

155   Natural Causes... Dan Hurley, *Natural Causes: Death, Lies and Politics in America's Vitamin and Herbal Supplement Industry* (New York: Broadway Books, 2006).

156   *"We did a study of Navy personnel"...* F. C. Garland, M. R. White, C. F. Garland, et al., "Occupational Sunlight Exposure and Melanoma in the U.S. Navy," *Archives of Environmental Health* 45, no. 5 (September–October 1990): 261–67.

157   *sunburn and high intermittent sun exposure actually increased the chances...* M. Berwick, B. K. Armstrong, L. Ben-Porat, et al., "Sun Exposure and Mortality from Melanoma," *Journal of the National Cancer Institute* 97 (2005): 195–99.

157   *At the 2005 American Association for Cancer Research meeting...* Associated Press, "Too Little Sun as Bad as Too Much? Scientists Say Vitamin D from Ultraviolet Rays May Fight Cancer," May 23, 2005, *www.msnbc.msn.com/ID/7875140/.* (Accessed on July 29, 2009.)

158   *deficiency of the vitamin early in life more than doubles the likelihood...* A. Giulietti, C. Gysemans, K. Stoffels, et al., "Vitamin D Deficiency in Early Life Accelerates Type 1 Diabetes in Non-obese Diabetic Mice," *Diabetologia* 47, no. 3 (March 2004): 451–62.

158   *mice given extra vitamin D had just one-seventh the risk ...* C. Mathieu, M. Waer, J. Laureys, et al., "Prevention of Autoimmune Diabetes in NOD Mice by 1,25 Dihydroxyvitamin D3," *Diabetologia* 37 (1994): 552–58.

158   *Bouillon wrote in 2002...* Chantal Mathieu, Evelyne van Etten, Conny Gysemans, et al., "Seasonality of Birth in Patients with Type 1 Diabetes," *Lancet*, 359, no. 9313 (April 6, 2002): 1248.

CHAPTER 9: THE HYGIENE HYPOTHESIS

Page

162 *John E. Craighead and Mary F. McLane...* J. E. Craighead and M. F. McLane, "Diabetes Mellitus: Induction in Mice by Encephalomyocarditis Virus," *Science* 162, no. 856 (November 22, 1968): 913–14.

162 *in 1969, a British group reported...* D. R. Gamble, M. L. Kinsley, and M. G. FitzGerald, "Viral Antibodies in Diabetes Mellitus," *British Medical Journal* 3 (September 13, 1969): 627–30.

162 The Lancet *published an editorial...* J. H. Karam, G. M. Grodsky, and P. H. Forsham, "Coxsackie Viruses and Diabetes," *Lancet* 2, no. 7735 (November 27, 1971): 1209.

162 *British Journal Says Tests Hint...* Lawrence K. Altman, "British Journal Says Tests Hint Diabetes May Be Caused by One or More Viruses," *New York Times*, October 29, 1971, page 20.

162 *In 1979, Dr. Ji-Won Yoon...* J. W. Yoon, M. Austin, and T. Onodera, "Isolation of a Virus from the Pancreas of a Child with Diabetic Ketoacidosis," *New England Journal of Medicine* 300, no. 21 (May 14, 1979): 1173–79.

162 *Close to half of the U.S. population had been exposed at some time in their lives to Coxsackie B4, yet less than 1 in 1,000 at that time had type 1 diabetes...* Harold M. Schmeck Jr., "Virus Link Is Found in Diabetes Patient," *New York Times*, May 24, 1979, page A1.

163 *A study in Erie County...* Nancy Hicks, "New Study Links Mumps, Diabetes," *New York Times*, October 23, 1974, page 17.

163 *Allegheny County, Pennsylvania, had a cluster...* T. M. Dokheel, "An Epidemic of Childhood Diabetes in the United States? Evidence from Allegheny County, Pennsylvania. Pittsburgh Diabetes Epidemiology Research Group," *Diabetes Care* 16, no. 2 (December 1993): 1606–1611.

163 *Birmingham, Alabama, had one linked to Coxsackie B5...* Lynne E. Wagenknecht, Jeffrey M. Roseman, and William H. Herman, "Increased Incidence of Insulin-Dependent Diabetes Mellitus Following an Epidemic of Coxsackievirus B5," *American Journal of Epidemiology* 133, no. 10 (1991): 1024–31.

163 *Philadelphia's 1993 uptick...* Terri H. Lipman, Yuefang Chang, and Kathryn M. Murphy, "The Epidemiology of Type 1 Diabetes in Children in Philadelphia 1990–1994: Evidence of an Epidemic," *Diabetes Care* 25 (2002): 1969–75.

163 *In 1676, when Antonie van Leeuwenhoek...* C. Dobell, *Anthony van Leeuwenhoek and His "Little Animals"* (New York: Russell & Russell, 1958).

164 *In 1963, neurologist David C. Poskanzer...* D. C. Poskanzer., K. Schapira, and H. Miller, "Multiple Sclerosis and Poliomyelitis," *Lancet* 2 (1963): 917–21.

164   *Uri Leibowitz and colleagues...* U. Leibowitz, A. Antonovsky, J. M. Medalie, et al., "Epidemiological Study of Multiple Sclerosis in Israel. II: Multiple Sclerosis and Level of Sanitation," *Journal of Neurology, Neurosurgery and Psychiatry* 29, no. 1 (February 1966): 60–68.

164   *613-word paper published in the* British Medical Journal... David P. Strachan, "Hay Fever, Hygiene, and Household Size," *British Medical Journal* 299 (1989): 1259–60.

166   *A 2008 study he co-authored...* C. R. Cardwell, L. C. Stene, G. Joner, et al., "Caesarean Section Is Associated with an Increased Risk of Childhood-Onset Type 1 Diabetes Mellitus: A Meta-Analysis of Observational Studies," *Diabetologia* 51, no. 5 (May 2008): 726–35.

166   *Another showed that children born in remote areas...* C. R. Cardwell, D. J. Carson, and C. C. Patterson, "Higher Incidence of Childhood-Onset Type 1 Diabetes Mellitus in Remote Areas: A UK Regional Small-Area Analysis," *Diabetologia* 49, no. 9 (September 2006): 2074–77.

166   *a third found that firstborn children are at increased risk...* C. R. Cardwell, D. J. Carson, and C. C. Patterson, "Parental Age at Delivery, Birth Order, Birth Weight and Gestational Age Are Associated with the Risk of Childhood Type 1 Diabetes: A UK Regional Retrospective Cohort Study," *Diabetic Medicine* 22, no. 2 (February 2005): 200–206.

166   *children with few infections in their first year...* C. R. Cardwell, D. J. Carson, and C. C. Patterson, "No Association Between Routinely Recorded Infections in Early Life and Subsequent Risk of Childhood-Onset Type 1 Diabetes," *Diabetic Medicine* 25, no. 3 (March 2008): 261–67.

166   *One of the first such studies, published in 1990...* M. W. Sadelain, H. Y. Qin, J. Lauzon, et al., "Prevention of Type I Diabetes in NOD Mice by Adjuvant Immunotherapy," *Diabetes* 39, no. 5 (May 1990): 583–89.

166   *In 2002, Japanese researchers...* H. Nomaguchi, Y. Yogi, K. Kawatsu, et al., "Prevention of Diabetes in Non-obese Diabetic Mice by a Single Immunization with Mycobacterium Leprae," *Nihon Hansenbyo Gakkai Zasshi* 71, no. 1 (February 2002): 31–38.

166   *Italian researchers reported...* F. Calcinaro, S. Dionisi, and M. Marinaro, "Oral Probiotic Administration Induces Interleukin-10 Production and Prevents Spontaneous Autoimmune Diabetes in the Non-obese Diabetic Mouse," *Diabetologia* 48, no. 8 (August 2005): 1565–75.

167   *French researchers reported...* M. A. Alyanakian, F. Grela, and A. Aumeunier, "Transforming Growth Factor-Beta and Natural Killer T-Cells Are Involved in the Protective Effect of a Bacterial Extract on Type 1 Diabetes," *Diabetes* 55, no. 1 (January 2006): 179–85.

167 *a truly beautiful study was published...* Li Wen, Ruth E. Ley, Pavel Y. Volch-kov, et al., "Innate Immunity and Intestinal Microbiota in the Development of Type 1 Diabetes," *Nature* 455, no. 7216 (October 23, 2008): 1109–1113.

168 *the immune systems of some wild wood mice...* J. M. Behnke, C. Eira, and M. Rogan, "Helminth Species Richness in Wild Wood Mice, Apodemus Sylvaticus, Is Enhanced by the Presence of the Intestinal Nematode Helig-mosomoides Polygyrus," *Parasitology* 136, no. 7 (June 2009): 793–804.

170 *a photograph of a man pulling a thin...* http://ib.berkeley.edu/courses/ib116/. (Accessed on July 30, 2009.)

170 *Search on Wikipedia and you'll end up reading about* Onchocera volvulus... http://en.wikipedia.org/wiki/Onchocerciasis. (Accessed on July 30, 2009.)

170 *check out the study in the journal* Burns... O. Lapid, Y. Krieger, and T. Bern-stein, "Airway Obstruction by Ascaris, Roundworm in a Burned Child," *Burns* 25, no. 7 (November 1999): 673–75.

171 *In 2003, Elliott and Weinstock took the daring step...* R. W. Summers, D. E. Elliott, K. Qadir, et al., "Trichuris Suis Seems to Be Safe and Possibly Effec-tive in the Treatment of Inflammatory Bowel Disease," *American Journal of Gastroenterology* 98, no. 9 (September 2003): 2034–41.

171 *a larger study, involving 54 people...* R. W. Summers, D. E. Elliott, J. F. Urban Jr., et al., "Trichuris Suis Therapy for Active Ulcerative Colitis: A Random-ized Controlled Trial," *Gastroenterology* 128, no. 4 (April 2005): 825–32.

171 *Another study of* Trichuris *eggs has now been undertaken* ... John Fleming, JangEun Lee, Christopher Luzzio, et al., "A Phase 1 Trial of Probiotic Hel-minth Ova in Relapsing Remitting Multiple Sclerosis (RRMS)," Abstract P07.141, American Academy of Neurology 2009 annual meeting, http:// msdiagnosed.org/news.php?open=431. (Accessed on July 30, 2009.)

174 *The first clear proof that infection with a helminth...* A. Cooke, P. Tonks, F. M. Jones, et al., "Infection with *Schistosoma mansoni* Prevents Insulin Dependent Diabetes Mellitus in Non-obese Diabetic Mice," *Parasite Immu-nology* 21, no. 4 (1999): 169–76.

174 *In 2003, she showed that injecting soluble extracts...* P. Zaccone, Z. Fehérvári, F. M. Jones, et al., "Schistosoma Mansoni Antigens Modulate the Activity of the Innate Immune Response and Prevent Onset of Type 1 Diabetes," *European Journal of Immunology* 33, no. 5: 1439–49.

174 *In 2007 she found the same effect...* K. A. Saunders, T. Raine, A. Cooke, et al., "Inhibition of Autoimmune Type 1 Diabetes by Gastrointestinal Helminth Infection," *Infection and Immunity* 75, no. 1 (2007): 397–407.

174 *in April of 2009, she again prevented diabetes...* P. Zaccone, O. Burton, N. Miller, et al., "Schistosoma Mansoni Egg Antigens Induce Treg that Participate in Diabetes Prevention in NOD Mice," *European Journal of Immunology* 39, no. 4 (2009): 1098–1107.

176 *Environmental Determinants of Diabetes in the Young....* For more information on TEDDY, see *http://teddy.epi.usf.edu/.* (Accessed on July 30, 2009.)

CHAPTER 10: THE COMPUTER CURE

Page

181 Relatively few studies have been published in the medical literature on recent breakthroughs in the development of an artificial pancreas, primarily because many of these developments are being financed by commercial enterprises, which protect their information from disclosure. However, two articles of notes include A. J. Kowalski, "Can We Really Close the Loop and How Soon? Accelerating the Availability of an Artificial Pancreas: A Roadmap to Better Diabetes Outcomes," *Diabetes Technology and Therapeutics* 11, Suppl. 1 (June 2009): S113–S119; and B. P. Kovatchev, M. Breton, and C. D. Man, "In Silico Preclinical Trials: A Proof of Concept in Closed-Loop Control of Type 1 Diabetes," *Diabetes Technology and Therapeutics* 11, Suppl. 1 (June 2009): S113–S119. For an up-to-date collection of news stories on JDRF's Artificial Pancreas Project, see *www.jdrf.org/index.cfm?page_id=104576.* (Accessed on July 30, 2009.)

181 *In the world of diabetes research...* Terry Fiedler, "Next: An Artificial Pancreas; Medical Giant Medtronic Says that an Elusive Goal in Diabetes Care May Soon Be Within Reach," *Star Tribune,* March 10, 2002.

181 *In May of 2006, Aaron Kowalksi...* Anita Manning, "Diabetics Get High-Tech Help to Track Sugar," *USA Today,* May 21, 2006, *www.usatoday.com/tech/news/techinnovations/2006-05-21-diabetes-monitoring_x.htm.*

181 *In September of 2007, Jennifer Aspy...* David Templeton, "New Tools Make Managing Disease a Good Deal Easier, but a Cure Is Still Far Off," *Pittsburgh Post-Gazette,* September 23, 2007, *www.post-gazette.com/pg/07266/819881-398.stm.*

184 *Tamborlane and his colleagues published...* W. V. Tamborlane, R. S. Sherwin, M. Genel, et al., "Reduction to Normal of Plasma Glucose in Juvenile Diabetes by Subcutaneous Administration of Insulin with a Portable Infusion Pump," *New England Journal of Medicine* 300, no. 11 (March 15, 1979): 573–78.

204 *I felt like the cognitively challenged guy...* Daniel Keyes, *Flowers for Algernon* (New York: Harcourt, 1966).

204 *on June 6, 2009, Medtronic announced...* See press release "Medtronic High-lights New Advances in Development of Closed-Loop System for Diabetes Management," *wwwp.medtronic.com/Newsroom/NewsReleaseDetails.do? itemId=1244301588079&lang=en_US.* (Accessed on July 30, 2009.)

204 *SmartInsulin...* See *www.smartinsulin.com.* For a PowerPoint presentation, see Todd C. Zion, "An Introduction to SmartInsulin," April 6, 2009, *www .slideshare.net/BringingTheCureHome/powerpoint-presentation-2-1319001.*

CHAPTER 11: THE SURGICAL CURE

Page

208 *"I want to win! I'm going to win,"...* Associated Press, "Clifton Oyster Shucker to Compete in Finland," *The Record,* April 7, 1992.

208 *"I expected to play in the Little League finals"...* Linda H. Burgess, "His Open-ing Act Was a Hit," *The Record,* May 13, 1992.

209 *he caught a* 60 Minutes *episode...* "The Bypass Effect on Diabetes, Cancer," April 20, 2008, *www.cbsnews.com/stories/2008/04/17/60minutes/main4023451. shtml.* (Accessed on July 31, 2009.)

209 *dubious medical "breakthroughs"—like shark cartilage...* See Dan Hurley, *Natural Causes: Death, Lies and Politics in America's Vitamin and Herbal Supplement Industry* (New York: Broadway Books, 2006): 201–204.

210 *risk of death among 7,925 people who underwent gastric bypass...* Ted D. Adams, Richard E. Gress, Sherman C. Smith, et al., "Long-Term Mortality after Gastric Bypass Surgery," *New England Journal of Medicine* 357, no. 8 (August 23, 2007): 753–61.

210 *Australian researchers published a randomized trial...* John B. Dixon, Paul E. O'Brien, Julie Playfair, et al., "Adjustable Gastric Banding and Conventional Therapy for Type 2 Diabetes: A Randomized Controlled Trial," *Journal of the American Medical Association* 299, no. 3 (2008): 316–23.

210 *The results were impressive enough to draw an editorial...* "Surgical Treat-ment for Diabetes," *New York Times,* January 24, 2008.

211 *a "meta-analysis" analyzing 621 prior studies...* Henry Buchwald, Rhonda Estok, Kyle Fahrbach, et al., "Weight and Type 2 Diabetes after Bariatric Surgery: Systematic Review and Meta-analysis," *American Journal of Medi-cine* 122, no. 3 (March 2009): 248–56.

212 *A 2007 paper by Judith Korner...* Judith Korner, Marc Bessler, William Inab-net, et al., "Exaggerated GLP-1 and Blunted GIP Secretion Are Associated with Roux-en-Y Gastric Bypass but Not Adjustable Gastric Banding," *Surgery for Obesity and Related Diseases* 3, no. 6 (2007): 597–601.

212 *A 2008 paper by Wei-Jei Lee...* W. J. Lee, W. Wang, Y. C. Lee, et al., "Effect of Laparoscopic Mini-Gastric Bypass for Type 2 Diabetes Mellitus: Comparison of BMI>35 and <35 kg/m2," *Journal of Gastrointestinal Surgery* 12, no. 5 (May 2008): 945–52.

213 *EndoBarrier gastrointestinal liner...* Dan Hurley, "New Procedures Provide Clues to Surgery's Effect on Diabetes," *General Surgery News* 36, no. 3 (2009), *http://my.clevelandclinic.org/Documents/Bariatric_Surgery/GSNewsDiabetes%20curable.pdf.* (Accessed on July 31, 2009.)

220 *1995 paper in the* Annals of Surgery... W. J. Pories, M. S. Swanson, K. G. MacDonald, et al., "Who Would Have Thought It? An Operation Proves to Be the Most Effective Therapy for Adult-Onset Diabetes Mellitus," *Annals of Surgery* 222, no. 3 (1995): 339–52.

CHAPTER 12: THE BIOLOGICAL CURE

Page

229 *The segment, broadcast on Monday, November 17, 2008...* A copy of the video can be found at *www.icue.com/portal/site/iCue/flatview/?cuecard=39096.* (Accessed on July 31, 2009.)

230 *"This is a crazy day because this paper is coming out,"...* C. Louvet, G. L. Szot, J. Lang, et al., "Tyrosine Kinase Inhibitors Reverse Type 1 Diabetes in Nonobese Diabetic Mice," *Proceedings of the National Academy of Sciences* 105, no. 48 (December 2008), 18895–900.

231 *Featured on the cover of* Time *magazine...* Christine Gorman, "Why Gleevec Got Approved," *Time,* May 21, 2001.

231 *The Immune Tolerance Network...* *www.immunetolerance.org/public.* (Accessed on July 31, 2009.)

234 *The JDRF alone spends some $160 million...* "JDRF's Annual Global Diabetes Research Forum Focused on Science, Hope for Adults with Type 1 Diabetes," June 19, 2008, *www.medicalnewstoday.com/articles/111934.php.* (Accessed on July 31, 2009.)

234 *the American Cancer Society spent...* Gina Kolata, "Grant System Leads Cancer Researchers to Play It Safe," *New York Times,* June 27, 2009, *www.nytimes.com/2009/06/28/health/research/28cancer.html?_r=1&hp.* (Accessed on August 1, 2009.)

234 *As the first to ever claim, back in 2001...* S. Ryu, S. Kodama, K. Ryu, et al., "Reversal of Established Autoimmune Diabetes by Restoration of Endogenous Beta Cell Function," *Journal of Clinical Investigation* 108 (2001): 63–72.

235 *In 2006, three independent teams...* J. Nishio, J. L. Gaglia, S. E. Turvey, et al., "Islet Recovery and Reversal of Murine Type 1 Diabetes in the Absence of Any Infused Spleen Cell Contribution," *Science* 311 (2006): 1775–78. A. Suri, B. Calderon, T. J. Esparza, et al., "Immunological Reversal of Autoimmune Diabetes without Hematopoietic Replacement of Beta Cells," *Science* 311 (2006), 1778–80. A. S. Chong, J. Shen, J. Tao, et al., "Reversal of Diabetes in Non-obese Diabetic Mice without Spleen Cell-Derived Beta Cell Regeneration, *Science* 311 (2006): 1774–75.

235 *In August of 2008, Faustman published...* L. Ban, J. Zhang, L. Wang, et al., "Selective Death of Autoreactive T Cells in Human Diabetes by TNF or TNF Receptor 2 Agonism," *Proceedings of the National Academy of Sciences* 105, no. 36 (September 9, 2008): 13644–13649.

235 *duct cells in the pancreas can be prodded* ... A. Inada, C. Nienaber, H. Katsuta, et al., "Carbonic Anhydrase II-Positive Pancreatic Cells Are Progenitors for Both Endocrine and Exocrine Pancreas After Birth," *Proceedings of the National Academy of Sciences* 105, no. 50 (December 2008): 19915–19.

236 *In August of 2008, he reported success...* Qiao Zhou, Juliana Brown, Andrew Kanarek, et al., "In Vivo Reprogramming of Adult Pancreatic Exocrine Cells To ß-Cells," *Nature* 455: 627–32. Published online August 27, 2008.

239 French researcher, Lucienne Chatenoud... L. Chatenoud, E. Thervet, and J. Primo, "Anti-CD3 Antibody Induces Long-Term Remission of Overt Autoimmunity in Nonobese Diabetic Mice," *Proceedings of the National Academy of Sciences* 91, no. 1 (January 4, 1994): 123–27.

CHAPTER 13: THE PUBLIC HEALTH CURE

Page

248 *a recent study in the* Archives of Internal Medicine... Patricia S. Keenan, "Smoking and Weight Change After New Health Diagnoses in Older Adults," *Archives of Internal Medicine* 169, no. 3 (February 9, 2009): 237–42.

248 Mindless Eating... Brian Wansink, *Mindless Eating: Why We Eat More than We Think* (New York: Bantam, 2006).

249 *My favorite of Wansink's many studies...* Pierre Chandon and Brian Wansink, "The Biasing Health Halos of Fast Food Restaurant Health Claims: Lower Calorie Estimates and Higher Side-Dish Consumption Intentions," *Journal of Consumer Research* 34, no. 3. (October 2007): 301–14.

249 *a person's chances of becoming obese jumps by 57 percent...* Nicholas A. Christakis and James H. Fowler, "The Spread of Obesity in a Large Social Network over 32 Years," *New England Journal of Medicine* 357, no. 4 (July 26, 2007): 370–79.

253 *A Canadian study published in June of 2009...* John C. Spencer, Nicoleta Cutumisu, Joy Edwards, et al., "Relation between Local Food Environments and Obesity Among Adults," *BMC Public Health* 9 (June 18, 2009): 192, *www .biomedcentral.com/1471-2458/9/192/abstract.* (Accessed August 1, 2009.)

253 *Another study, presented at a recent meeting of the American Stroke Association...* Lewis B. Morgenstern, James D. Escoba, Rebecca Hughes, et al., "Number of Fast-Food Restaurants in Neighborhood Associated with Stroke Risk," Abstract P162 (February 16, 2009), *http://americanheart.mediaroom. com/index.php?s=43&item=666.* (Accessed August 1, 2009.)

253 *In Mississippi, for instance, State Representative John Read...* "The Smoking Gun: Mississippi Pols Seek to Ban Fats; New Bill Would Make It Illegal for Restaurants to Serve the Obese," February 1, 2008, *www.thesmokinggun .com/archive/years/2008/0201081fat1.html.* (Accessed August 1, 2009.)

253 *a bill proposed to place a one-year moratorium...* Karl Vick, "L.A. Official Wants a Change of Menu; Councilwoman Seeks Moratorium on New Fast-Food Restaurants in South-Central," *Washington Post,* July 13, 2008, page A2.

254 *a total ban on all TV commercials for fast-food restaurants...* Shin-Yi Chou, Inas Rashad, and Michael Grossman, "Fast-Food Restaurant Advertising on Television and Its Influence on Childhood Obesity," *Journal of Law and Economics* 51, no. 4 (November 2008): 599–618.

254 *Marion Nestle...* Marion Nestle, *Food Politics: How the Food Industry Influences Nutrition and Health* (Berkeley: University of California Press, 2002). Marion Nestle, *What to Eat: An Aisle by Aisle Guide to Savvy Food Choices and Good Eating* (New York: North Point Press, 2006).

254 *In Defense of Food...* Michael Pollan, *In Defense of Food: An Eater's Manifesto* (New York: Penguin Press, 2008).

255 *"Advice focused on individuals has not succeeded"...* Marion Nestle, "Preventing Childhood Diabetes: The Need for Public Health Intervention," *American Journal of Public Health* 95, no. 9 (September 2005): 1497–99.

255 *A ruling in favor of the restaurant association...* Ray Rivera, "Fight to Put Calories on Menus May Widen," *New York Times,* September 13, 2007, page B3.

256 *In response, Health Commissioner Thomas Frieden quipped...* Ibid.

256 *Judge Holwell ruled in favor of the Board...* James Barron, "Restaurants Must Post Calories, Judge Affirms," *New York Times,* April 17, 2008, page B4.

256 *New York City health inspectors soon went about...* James Barron, "5 Manhattan Restaurants Cited for Lack of Calorie Counts on Menu," *New York Times,* May 6, 2008, page B4.

256 *Way back in 1980, Kelly Brownell...* K. D. Brownell, A. J. Stunkard, and J. M. Albaum, "Evaluation and Modification of Exercise Patterns in the Natural Environment," *American Journal of Psychiatry* 137 (1980): 1540–45.

259 *according to the CDC's 2006 School Health Policies and Programs Study... www .cdc.gov/HealthyYouth/physicalactivity/facts.htm.* (Accessed on August 1, 2009.)

259 *article by Associated Press reporter Nancy Armour...* Nancy Armour, "PE Requirement Isn't Enough to Fight Obesity," June 15, 2009, *http://abcnews. go.com/Health/wireStory?id=7845836.* (Accessed on August 1, 2009.)

259 *only 23 percent of consumers surveyed by the health department...* The findings of this survey were sent as a personal communication to me from the New York City Department of Health and Mental Hygiene.

260 *"lifestyle tax proposals"...* Alan Fram, "The Influence Game: New Drink Tax Widely Opposed," June 3, 2009, *http://abcnews.go.com/Politics/ wireStory?id=7745754.* (Accessed on August 1, 2009.)

260 *Richard Daines became an unlikely YouTube sensation... www.youtube.com/ watch?v=ARMgjdbY930.* (Accessed on August 1, 2009.)

261 *"significant" federal funds...* Maggie Fox, "U.S. States to Get 'Significant' Obesity Money," Reuters, July 28, 2009, *www.reuters.com/article/domestic News/idUSTRE56R5UH20090728?feedType=RSS&feedName=domesticNews& rpc=22&sp=true.* (Accessed on August 3, 2009.)

261 *a federal appellate court rejected it...* New York State Restaurant Assoc. v. New York City Board of Health, No. 08-1892-cv (2d Cir. Feb. 17, 2009), decision available at *www.citizen.org/documents/NYSRAOpinion.pdf.* (Accessed on August 1, 2009.)

CONCLUSION

Page

264 *in 2006, there were 72,507 death certificates...* Centers for Disease Control and Prevention, 2007 National Diabetes Fact Sheet, *www.cdc.gov/diabetes/pubs/ estimates07.htm.* (Accessed on August 1, 2009.)

264 *America's 23 million people with diabetes...* Ibid.

INDEX

Index

O

Obama, President, 261
Obesity, 8, 94, 249
O'Connell, Chris, 204
OM-85 bacterial extract, 167
Omnipod pump, 199
Onchocera volvulus, 170
O'Neill, Brendan, xviii
O'Neill, Melissa, xviii
Ooten, Sandra, 82–83
Opium, 7, 11
Orinase, 36–40, 69
Ortiz, David, xiii
Ovamed GmbH, 172, 173
Overture, 185, 186

P

Pablum, 121
Pallozzi-Haynes, Tom, 207–10, 213–16,
    224–27
Palmer, MD, Jerry P., 102
Pancreas, x, 10
    artificial, 181–205
Pancreatic extract. 13–14
Pancreatic pain receptors, 125
Paradigm Real-Time, 53–56
Pasteur, Louis, 164
Patek, PhD, Steven, 203
Pediatrics, 151
Peninsula Medical School, 91
Perchloroethylene (PCE), 127, 132–35, 143
Pergams, Oliver, 151
Perry, Jan, 254
"Persistent organic pollutants" (POPs),
    135–38, 139–41, 142
Pfizer & Co., 37
Pharmaceutice Rationalis, 5
Phenformin, 37–38, 40, 69
Philadelphia *Inquirer,* 257
Physical exercise, 25
Pill, first, 34–36
Pi-Sunyer, MD, F. Xavier, 211
Pittsburgh *Post-Gazette,* 181
Plaque buildup, 30
Plaza's Oyster Bar, 208
"Pogo," 42

Polio, 245
Pollan, Michael, 254
Polychlorinated biphenyls (PCBs), 134–35,
    136, 141
Polychlorinated dibenzofurans (PCDFs), 134
Pooler, Rosemary S., 261
Pories, MD, Walter J., 220
Poskanzer, David C., 164
Prameha, 5
Prescribing by Numbers, 37, 39
Pro-biotic, 166–67
*Proceedings of the National Academy of
    Sciences,* 151, 235, 243
Prograf, 58
Protamine, 34
Protamine zinc insulin, 35
Protein
    foreign, 119–21
    intake, 110–11
Public Citizen, 41
Public health, 245–61

Q–R

Queen's University of Belfast, 166
Quinaretic, 67
Rapamune, 58
Read, John, 253
Record, 208
Restani, Jane A., 261
Retinitis, 30
Retinopathy, 76
Rezulin, 70–71
Rice-bran oil, 134
Richard, Kathy, xvii
Richard, Sean, xv, xvii
Roach, Edith, 14, 20
Robinson, Jackie, 42
Roche Diabetes Care, 181, 192
Roglic, MD, Gojka, xxii, 222–23
Rollo, John, 6–7, 8
Rosenbloom, MD, Alran, 149
Roux-En-Y procedure, 212, 214–15
Rubino, MD, Francesco, 209–10, 211,
    214–19, 221–23, 226
Rudd Center for Food Policy and
    Obesity, 248

309